Essential Exercises
for Breast Cancer Survivors

Essential Exercises
for Breast Cancer Survivors

Amy Halverstadt and Andrea Leonard

The Harvard Common Press
Boston, Massachusetts

The Harvard Common Press
535 Albany Street
Boston, Massachusetts 02118

Printed in the United States of America
Printed on acid-free paper

Library of Congress Cataloging-in-Publication Data

Halverstadt, Amy.

    Essential exercises for breast cancer survivors : how to live stronger and feel better /
Amy Halverstadt and Andrea Leonard ; foreword by Peggy Fleming ; introduction by Shawna C. Willey.
        p.   cm.
    Includes bibliographical references and index.
    ISBN 1-55832-178-0 (hc : alk. paper) — ISBN 1-55832-179-9 (pbk. : alk. paper)
    1. Breast—Cancer—Exercise therapy. 2. Exercise for women. I. Leonard, Andrea. II. Title.

RC280.B8 H357 2000
616.99'449062—dc21   00-040719

Cover design by Night & Day Design
Photographs by John Gillooly
Illustrations by Elizabeth Morales
Production by Eclipse Publishing Services

10 9 8 7 6 5 4 3 2 1

To Andrea Leonard's mother, Edythe Beres, whose courage and strength in the face of her lengthy breast cancer challenge provided the inspiration for this book;

To Amy Halverstadt's close friends who have faced the challenges of breast cancer and continue the fight against this disease;

To Marlene Haffner, Francesca Danielli, Jessica Einhorn, Anne Gurvin, Bonnie Goldstein, and Katherine Anthony, who are living proof that fortitude and willpower are better companions than fear and negativity; and

To those whose lives are impacted by breast cancer as survivors, friends, and relatives.

WE HOPE this book helps you and those you love lead fuller lives.

Contents

Foreword

FOR ME AS A YOUNG GIRL, exercise strengthened not only my body, it also strengthened my soul. As I gained stamina, muscle, and balance, I also gained a confidence that would make me more resilient to life's challenges.

In 1998, when I was diagnosed with breast cancer, I once again turned to that early tool of measuring myself through exercise. Throughout my treatment and recovery, I would gently test myself physically to see how I was doing. Small steps led to bigger ones, and each success at exercise reassured me that I was going to be OK—that I was still me. Today I'm back to feeling like myself. It just took time and patience.

A health crisis can be a real test to your character, but in facing that crisis you may just find a strength you never knew you had. Who knows—with this book's guidance you may also find out that exercise is fun!

I hope that exercise will help you find the power that really is inside each of us, and that *Essential Exercises for Breast Cancer Survivors* will help guide you back to health and to the person you may have thought you lost.

Peggy Fleming Jenkins

Acknowledgments

THE AUTHORS would like to thank the many people who have contributed their time, expertise, and experiences to make this book a reality. Without them, it would not have been possible. A special thank-you goes to Shawna Willey, M.D.; Marlene Haffner, M.D.; Theodore Tsiangaris Jr., M.D.; and Jean Lynn, RN, BS, OCN. These professionals dedicated their time and expertise to ensuring the accuracy and thoroughness of this book. A special thank-you also goes to Dana Phares, M.A., and Rosalie Begun, P.T., for their time and expertise, their dedication to improving women's health and quality of life, and for their support and direction not only of this project but of other projects focused on enhancing the lives of breast cancer survivors.

In addition, we would like to thank Edythe Beres; Marlene Haffner, M.D.; Jessica Einhorn; Anne Gurvin; Francesca Danielli; Bonnie Goldstein; and Katherine Anthony. These breast cancer survivors dedicated their time and serve as the hope and inspiration for the book.

We would like to thank Steven Fay and Scott Leonard for their support, guidance, unending patience, insight, and experience.

A special thank-you goes to Donna Halverstadt, Sandi Wilson, Clare Donaher, and Annie Groer for their critical support and unending belief in this project; to Kevin Fay and Grace Lawson for their invaluable time, counsel, and expertise; to Anita Brienza for unselfishly giving her time, insight, and expertise; to Ann Saybolt for her time; to Sumter Brawley for his graciousness, faith, and dedication; and to Jed Lyons for his belief and support.

Finally, we want to express our heartfelt gratitude and love for our parents and families—Donald, Peggy, Donna, and Jeff Halverstadt, and Morton, Edythe, and Keith Beres—for being exceptional mentors and for giving their love and support unconditionally.

Introduction

Shawna C. Willey, M.D. FACS
Chief of Breast Surgery
The George Washington University Medical Center

WOMEN WHO HAVE HAD SURGERY for breast cancer have concerns that their lives will be changed forever (they will) and that they will be disabled by the surgery (they won't). What is surprising to most women is that there should be no physical limitations after breast surgery and that they can expect to regain full mobility, control, and stamina. This book is a tool to make sure that happens.

One of the questions posed to me most frequently during a post-operative appointment with breast cancer patients is "When can I exercise?". I first met Amy and Andrea when they approached me about enrolling patients in an exercise program they had developed for women who had recently or even long ago undergone surgery for breast cancer. I realized that, although I was a big proponent of getting patients moving and returning to their usual activities after surgery, I was not particularly knowledgeable about the limitations I should place on their exercise. I did not feel well-versed in counseling and advising patients about proper exercise technique or which activities to avoid. I had only my personal experience from talking to hundreds of women about the benefits of their exercise programs and some of the problems they had encountered with them. The program that Amy and Andrea have developed is the culmination of years of work with breast cancer survivors, as well as Amy's and Andrea's personal experiences of breast cancer touching their lives. *Essential Exercises for Breast Cancer Survivors* tells you how to start a sensible, safe, lifetime exercise program.

It's important to remember that this program should be tailored to your individual needs. Just as your breast cancer treatment was designed specifically for you so that you received, for example, the right amount of radiation or the correct dose of chemotherapy, so should this program evolve to match your specific exercise needs and limitations. If you've ever attended a support group, you know how varied the reaction can be to a treatment or even to a statement by a health care provider. So, too, in the exercise world. Throughout the book there are many suggestions as to how to individualize your program. *Essential Exercises* outlines a standard set of exercises in a specific pattern, but finding the proper "FITT" is up to you. (You'll learn about that term in Chapter 5.)

Being diagnosed and treated for breast cancer is a life-altering event for all women. All of us (yes, even surgeons) wonder how we would respond to being told we have breast cancer. The words "You have cancer" instantly change your world. The reassurance all women seek is that they will survive. The statistics for survival from breast cancer are good compared with many other kinds of malignancies. But the initial fears that "I won't see Christmas," "I won't see my son's graduation," "I must be here for my daughter" give way to a more rational response as a woman learns about her stage of disease, treatment, and her own personal survival statistics. Breast cancer isn't fair or predictable. As many as 75 percent of women diagnosed with breast cancer have no known risk factor for the development of this disease. Women want to be reassured that at some point life will be "normal" again. This book can help you with that normalization process during and after therapy.

The whole breast cancer treatment experience is demoralizing. You have the pain and alteration in body image that goes with surgery. It is true that breast conservation and breast reconstruction have improved the degree of these alterations significantly, but even if you have a small scar on your breast with no significant change in appearance, there *is* an alteration in your body's appearance. If you've had chemotherapy, it's likely that you've lost some if not all of your hair. That's demoralizing! I've had very few patients who truly didn't mind being bald. Along with the chemotherapy go the nausea, the fatigue, joint aches, "chemo brain," worry about blood counts and staying on schedule. Radiation, along with the annoyance of requiring you to be there *every day,* adds to your fatigue and may change the way your breast feels or looks or alter your range of motion. The hormone treatment tamoxifen is well-tolerated, but it may have side effects you don't enjoy, like hot flashes and vaginal discharge. Many women who have been through any or all of these treatment regimens will notice weight gain, mood swings, loss of libido, or depression. Responses vary, but few women go through the whole experience unscathed by any of these problems. But there is life after breast cancer.

After I've operated on a woman for breast cancer, I generally refer her to a physical therapist within three to six weeks of surgery for an initial assessment of range of motion, lymphedema precaution instructions, and exercise education. If your surgeon has not offered that option to you, ask about it. Not all geographic areas have physical therapists experienced in working with breast cancer patients. If you live in an area that doesn't, find a physical therapist who is willing to learn about therapy specifically for breast cancer survivors and perhaps, with *Essential Exercises,* you can educate yourselves together. By being an advocate, you, and possibly those diagnosed after you, will benefit. The physical therapist you recruit may be someone you will need as a resource if any difficulties or questions arise during your exercise program.

When a woman has completed treatment, she faces the phase of "getting on with life." It's at this point that I see many women making a commitment to a healthier lifestyle and improving their self-image. Exercise is the key to that self-improvement plan. We all have plenty of excuses as to why we don't exercise. But there are even more barriers for the woman who has had breast cancer. There is a fear that the exercise might cause damage, that it could start lymphedema, that it's too soon after surgery for exercise, that it's too late to do any good, that she physically can't do the exercise, that she'll look funny, that she doesn't want to undress in front of people. (What's your excuse?) Exercise, even to a minimal degree, is beneficial, but especially for the breast cancer survivor who is putting behind her the treatment sequence and the sense of lack of control that goes with it. Exercise is an empowering activity. Look at all the Races and Walks for the Cure! There's a reason all those women are out there running and walking. Exercise is an option a woman has full control over, and it produces noticeable effects and benefits almost immediately. If you do it on a "buddy system" or in a class, it can become a support group for you. By picking up this book, you have made a statement that you are open to the concept of exercise. Hopefully, the authors will convince you that this is a good thing to do, that *you* can do it, and that you will benefit from it.

Essential Exercises for Breast Cancer Survivors outlines a series of exercises to take you from timid beginner to enthusiastic participant. A regimen that is progressive with measurable milestones will give you a sense of accomplishment and confidence. There are suggestions for a variety of activities, including choices for aerobic exercise as well as weight lifting. I hope this book will educate you and motivate you to become the active person you're destined to be. There *is* life after breast cancer. It's in your power to make it the best life that you can!

PART I

Exercise, Breast Cancer, and You

CHAPTER 1

Why Should I Exercise?

The beauty of the energy of exercise is that it unites all of the disparate parts of the body. I become myself again.

Anne Gurvin, Breast Cancer Survivor

There are no riches above a sound body. —Ecclesiasticus 30:16

THIS BOOK will take you on a journey. It will explain why you should exercise, how your treatment may affect your exercise program, how to begin exercising, how to continue and progress, and how to assess your progress. The goals of *Essential Exercises for Breast Cancer Survivors* are as follows:

- To enhance your energy level through physical activity
- To improve your posture by stretching tight muscles and strengthening weak ones
- To increase your range of motion through stretching and movement exercises (with an emphasis on the upper body)
- To strengthen the body's core stabilizers—the abdominal and lower back muscles—through targeted exercises and dynamic movement

- To improve your quality of life by enhancing your physical and mental condition through exercise training

This last point in particular means that although the program was designed as a postoperative workout, it is appropriate for all women and men living with breast cancer. Whether you were just diagnosed, are at least six weeks postoperative, or are at some other appropriate stage of treatment, *Essential Exercises* can help you build the power of your body and your mind.

Benefits of Exercise for Everyone

As part of the recipe for a better, healthier life, exercise can do some amazing things. It not only helps us control our weight and decrease our risk of disease, but it can also make us physically stronger, improve our psychological and emotional states, and keep us independent. Exercise can help you, as a breast cancer survivor, take back your life and look forward. It can help you live strong and take better care of yourself. Reaping these many benefits of exercise and reaching your physical and emotional potential are what this book is all about. *Essential Exercises for Breast Cancer Survivors* will show you how to add exercise to your own recipe for living stronger.

With all the information available on the benefits of exercise, and with our society's desire to be healthier, look better, and live longer for our families and ourselves, it's intriguing that most Americans shy away from exercise. Perhaps we feel too tired from our jobs, relationships, and kids to exercise. It's tempting at the end of a long day to sit back and order a pizza while watching television. That's a good time to remember what Will Rogers said: "Why not go out on a limb? That's where the fruit is!" By trying something new and challenging, we can enjoy new rewards. Incorporating more exercise into your life may be a bit difficult at first, but you will find that with a little time and perseverance, exercise becomes easier and more fun. Really!

At this point, you probably have lots of questions and concerns swirling around inside your head. For one thing, you may be asking yourself, "What kind of exercise can I do?" There are many avenues of exercise that can accommodate your various interests and responsibilities. In fact, a variety of exercise is a good idea. And exercising with other people can make it easier to get started. Get your family involved: Take your kids hiking, biking, or walking. Throw a ball, play hoops, or just dance around your living room. You may even find yourself enjoying exercise. Unbelievable? Wait and see!

What Exercise Does

- Helps maintain independence
- Helps lift your spirits and reduce feelings of depression
- Increases muscular strength and endurance and aerobic capacity
- Reduces body fat and improves body composition
- Assists in weight management and weight loss
- Improves feelings of self-confidence and control
- Makes everyday tasks easier and more enjoyable
- Reduces the risks of illnesses such as diabetes, obesity, heart disease, high blood pressure, osteoarthritis, osteoporosis, and certain cancers

For starters, don't worry that you don't have time in your busy schedule. Keep in mind that anything you do, any progress you make, is better than doing nothing at all. You may feel uncomfortable going to a gym. You are not alone. For many of us, going to a gym is extremely intimidating. You walk into a mirrored room filled with muscle-bound men and women grunting and groaning as they lift enormous dumbbells and flex their bulging biceps. Maybe the neon lights are flashing and the music is blasting, and here you are facing machines that look like something out of a *Star Wars* movie, without a single clue as to how to use them. Entering this unfamiliar environment is a difficult task even for most people who haven't gone through the traumatic surgery you have. With an altered body image and freshly healing wounds, the last thing you need is to feel uncomfortable in a new social situation. *Essential Exercises for Breast Cancer Survivors* can help you get started and feel comfortable with your own exercise program. That, in turn, can make you more confident about exercising regularly and in different settings.

Benefits of Exercise for Breast Cancer Survivors

As a breast cancer survivor, you probably have undergone some intense medical treatment and rehabilitation: surgery, radiation, drugs, and basic physical therapy (hopefully, you were prescribed physical therapy or given basic therapeutic exercises after treatment). Maybe you also got involved with a support group or organization that helped you in your recovery. But what about the next step—taking the strengthening of your body and mind to another level and becoming physically and emotionally stronger than you were before your diagnosis and treatment? *Essential Exercises for Breast Cancer Survivors* embodies just that concept—taking control of your life from here forward, treating your whole person and not just the disease, and becoming stronger as a result of your experiences. As a physical reconditioning program developed specifically for breast cancer survivors and based on the experiences of other survivors just like you, *Essential Exercises* will help you rebuild your strength, self-esteem, and self-confidence through exercise.

Although we talk about the general importance of exercise, the bottom line is that *Essential Exercises* is about you and your individual goals. While reading through this book, you may feel that you are being made to face yet another challenge in addition to breast cancer—that of incorporating exercise into your life. It may make you feel more at ease to know that many others are starting on this path with you. Like them, you may reap the many rewards that come with regular exercise.

The Facts

You've already experienced breast cancer, and you can't change your past. But the information that is becoming available about the role of exercise and eating right in the prevention of breast cancer is worth talking about. In regard to exercise, two studies highlight the role exercise can play in reducing the risk of breast cancer. Researchers at the University of Southern California found that women under forty who exercised four or more hours per week during their reproductive years had almost a 60 percent lower risk of getting breast cancer than inactive women. Researchers in Norway found that women who exercised at least four hours per week reduced their risk of breast cancer by 37 percent, as compared with sedentary women. In regular exercisers, risk reduction was greater in women who were under age forty-five, women who were lean and exercised at least four hours per week, and women who had been regular exercisers for three to five years. A 1997 report by the American Institute for Cancer Research outlines evidence about the role of nutrition in the prevention of cancer. It concludes that, in addition to exercise, a healthy, low-fat, high-fiber diet may reduce the risk of breast cancer, as well as other diseases.

The evidence is clear: exercise regularly and reduce the amount of fat in your diet, and you may give yourself a longer, healthier, more productive life.

Although we often view exercise and diet as a means to look good, we should remember that it plays a major role in our health. True, we want to be able to put on our jeans without having to lie down on the bed and hold our breath to pull up the zipper, but we should also want to be healthy and feel good. When viewed in relation to breast cancer, exercise and nutrition take on a much larger meaning than just that snug piece of denim.

Cancer, Exercise, and Self-Expression

Unlike the flu or the common cold, you don't feel cancer coming on. By the time you hear those awful words "You have cancer," the disease has already invaded your body. There are rarely clear warning signs, and you can't get well by taking extra vitamin C or sleeping it off under a warm down comforter. Not only are you faced with a life-threatening illness, but you have to make some quick decisions about treatment that will move your life in a direction you never anticipated. In some ways, your life is out of your hands and may seem out of control. Nothing can take away the shock and fear of discovering that you have breast cancer, but exercise can do something significant for you: it can help you regain the feeling of being in control of your life, your body, and your destiny.

Think of exercise as your secret weapon against the possible physical and psychological impact of breast cancer diagnosis and treatment. Physically, you may find that you have lost strength and mobility in your affected arm and shoulder, you may have lost bone density, you may be nauseous, and you may just be totally worn-out. Emotionally, you may be drained, depressed, and frustrated. Good news: moderate physical activity can help counter many of these effects. Exercise—your secret weapon—can help you do the following:

- Avoid the physical side effects caused by bed rest, such as decreased muscle strength and endurance
- Regain strength and mobility in your arms and shoulders
- Increase your ability to perform daily activities without becoming fatigued
- Reduce anxiety and depression and improve your overall sense of well-being

You can also think of exercise as a means of self-expression. Cancer is unfair. It's sneaky, it cheats us, and it deserves a good pop in the nose—and you deserve a way to give it one. By choosing activities that you enjoy and participating at your own pace, you express your own creativity and drive to win the battle against cancer. You show yourself and the world your inner strength and courage. You embark on the path to a better quality of life.

Benefits of Exercise for You

Essential Exercises for Breast Cancer Survivors is about helping you start or continue your own exercise program. As with any exercise program, *you must get approval from your doctor before you begin.*

Essential Exercises shows you how you can exercise at various levels in the comfort of your own home. No fancy equipment is required, and you can choose how much time you want to dedicate to exercising. We make suggestions as to how often, how long, and at what intensity you should exercise. You choose your own pace. Be persistent and be proud of the changes you're making. At times you may feel like giving up, especially if you feel minor discomfort. But go slowly and just keep trying. If you're frustrated with a particular exercise, move on to the next and try the difficult one at another time. If you're still frustrated, take a break and think of all the good you're doing for yourself. If you belong to a support group, call an exercise buddy; if not, call a friend for some encouragement. But, most important, remember that you are taking control and building a stronger you.

In case you need further encouragement to begin to exercise, following is a recap of some of the many physiological, psychological, and other benefits of a regular exercise program.

Physiological Benefits of Regular Exercise
- Improved aerobic endurance and physical stamina (stronger heart and lungs)
- Increased muscular strength and endurance
- Improved body composition (less fat, more muscle)
- Reduced blood pressure
- Increased metabolic rate (Building muscle can increase your body's calorie-burning rate and help you lose weight or maintain weight loss.)
- Increased high-density lipoprotein (HDL) cholesterol (the "good" cholesterol)
- Decreased risk of diseases such as coronary artery disease, diabetes, obesity, hypertension, high cholesterol, and osteoporosis

Affirmations

Tell yourself that you are beautiful, strong, and a survivor. Don't let any-one tell you that you cannot or should not exercise—unless, of course, it is your doctor. And, most important, remember that you are doing this because it is one of the best gifts you can give yourself.

Try the following affirmations to keep yourself motivated.

- Exercise may possibly help me reduce my chances of getting cancer again.

- Exercise can help me regain the feeling of controlling my life, my body, and my destiny; can increase strength and mobility in my arms and shoulders; and can improve my ability to perform daily activities without becoming fatigued.

- I can make my life better by choosing to do something that may be a little difficult and challenging for me.

- I have already faced one of the hardest things in life, and I survived. I can handle a little exercise.

Psychological Benefits of Regular Exercise
- Decreased stress and tension
- Increased self-esteem and self-confidence
- Increased ability to concentrate and cope with stressors
- Improved feeling of general well-being and reduced anxiety and depression

Other Benefits of Regular Exercise
- Improved cancer treatment tolerance (for instance, less nausea and fatigue)
- Improved sleep
- Improved muscle tone (physical appearance)
- Increased group support or personal time

CHAPTER 2

Treatment and Exercise

Surgery, radiation, and chemotherapy can have extensive effects on body strength and self-esteem. Exercise is an affirmation that your body still belongs to you and can be a source of joy through unrestrained motion, increased strength and graceful flexibility. Physically and psychologically, exercise was crucial to my getting through treatment and on the road to recovery.

Jessica Einhorn

You gain strength, courage, and confidence by every experience in which you really stop to look fear in the face. . . . You must do the things you cannot do. —*Eleanor Roosevelt*

To UNDERSTAND HOW *Essential Exercises for Breast Cancer Survivors* can help you rebuild strength and relieve pain after treatment for breast cancer, we need to review the anatomy of the breast and the lymphatic system, breast cancer itself, and the various treatments for the disease. This chapter provides that overview. It also reviews the potential side effects associated with each treatment and discusses how treatment can affect your exercise program.

This material may be difficult for you to read because you may not want to relive your cancer and its treatment. Some of the discussion is a bit technical in nature. But knowledge is power, and power—to improve your physical and mental condition after breast cancer treatment—is what this program is all about.

If you want more information on the disease and treatments, talk with your medical care providers, or see the resources and references sections in the back of this book.

The Disease

Cancer can be described as a disease in which abnormal (malignant) cells divide and form additional abnormal cells without any order or control. The problem with these malignant cells is that they are unable to perform the functions they were designed for—such as to replace worn-out cells or repair damaged cells—and they can continue to grow and multiply without constraint. The abnormal cells do not respond appropriately to the body's signals to divide only when needed and to stop when that need is fulfilled. In other words, these cells can be thought of as taking on a life of their own. A tumor is formed when millions of these cells have divided and grown in one place. The cells can invade and destroy healthy tissue and can spread and grow in other areas of the body.

How does this happen? What causes an abnormal cell? Although these questions have yet to be answered completely, scientists do know that the DNA (genetic code) of these abnormal cells has in some way been damaged (although not all cells with damaged DNA become cancerous). Scientists know of three ways this can happen: some type of mistake is made in the normal cell division process; factors outside the cell or the body cause damage to the DNA; or damaged DNA is inherited. For cells with damaged DNA to become cancer cells, the body's own control system must fail. That is, specific genes that are designed to look for damaged DNA and stop its production do not do so. The damaged cells are then able to divide without control.

When these abnormal, cancerous cells are found in the breast, the disease is called breast cancer. If breast cancer cells spread and invade other parts of the body, the disease is still breast cancer because the invading cells are abnormal breast cells. As with all cancers, this process begins with just one cell. In breast cancer, the disease usually starts as a single cell in the ducts or lobules. It usually takes place there because that is where periods of rapid cell division and growth occur during the different phases of the menstrual cycle. It is important to note that the body signals the increase in cell division by way of two hormones, estrogen and progesterone. Knowing that these hormones may be a signal for both normal and cancerous breast cell growth and division will help you understand some of the treatment and guidance you may receive. One breast cell with damaged DNA may respond to the production of estrogen and progesterone by growing and dividing, then fail to respond to the body's signal to stop dividing. Once this process has started and the cancer is growing, it can take months or years before there is a mass of cells, or a tumor, big enough to cause symptoms or to be detected by touch or X ray.

Breast Anatomy and the Lymphatic System

The breasts are mammary glands, which secrete milk. The glandular tissue of the breasts lies over two main muscles—the large chest muscle (pectoralis major) and one of the shoulder girdle muscles (serratus anterior)—and covers the area from the armpit to the breastbone (sternum) and from the second to the sixth rib. Each breast is composed of fifteen to twenty sections called lobes, which consist of smaller sections called lobules. These lobules are groups of individual milk glands. Within each lobe, there is a system of branching ducts, or small tubes, which transport milk produced by the lobules within it. These branching ducts join together to form larger ducts, which then empty the milk into the nipple. The tissue surrounding the lobes consists of fat and connective tissue, which provide form, shape, and support for the breast.

The lymphatic system is one of the body's eleven organ systems. Its main functions include the following:

- Aids the immune system in protecting the body from disease
- Returns fluids to the blood in the circulatory system
- Transports fat from the digestive tract to the blood
- Produces blood cells
- Filters bacteria, viruses, tissue debris, and other foreign substances from body fluids

The lymphatic system is made up of vessels, fluid, and nodes. Lymph vessels form a network that runs throughout the body. Similar to the ducts in the breast, lymph vessels are transport tubes that carry, or drain, fluid from the surrounding tissue. Once in the lymphatic vessels, this fluid is called lymph. The lymphatic vessels return this fluid to the blood by draining into the large veins close to the heart. Along the lymph vessels are small, kidney-shaped masses called lymph nodes. These lymph nodes filter debris and other foreign material, such as cancer cells, from the lymph fluid. Sometimes these nodes are clustered in certain areas of the body and are named for the area in which they are found. Breast cancer patients are most interested in the clusters of nodes in the armpit (axillary nodes), under the clavicle or collarbone (supraclavicular nodes), and alongside the sternum (parasternal or internal mammary nodes).

The lymph fluid from a certain region of the body flows through the nodes found in the same region. Thus, fluid from the breast area flows through the clusters of nodes mentioned in the previous paragraph. If cancer cells have spread, some may be trapped in the lymph nodes. This is why the lymph nodes are examined to help determine whether the cancer has spread outside the breast.

Breast Cancer: Types and Locations

There are several types of breast cancer, and cancer can be found in different areas of the breast. Generally, the cancer can be noninvasive (in situ) or invasive (infiltrating) and can begin in the cells lining the ducts (ductal carcinoma) or the lobules (lobular carcinoma). Most commonly, breast cancer begins in one of the cells lining the ducts.

If a cancer is noninvasive, or in situ, it has not spread to areas outside the ducts or lobules. If it is invasive, or infiltrating, it has penetrated the ductal or lobular walls and spread to the surrounding tissue. The spread of cancer can also be said to be local or regional or to have formed a distant metastasis. Local or regional cancer has spread into the surrounding tissue or lymph nodes. Metastasis means that the disease has spread from where it started to other areas of the body. Breast cancer metastases can affect areas such as the lungs, liver, bones, or brain.

Following are some of the main categories of breast cancer.

Infiltrating Ductal Carcinoma

This is the most common type of breast cancer and accounts for 65 to 85 percent of cases. This cancer starts in the cells lining the wall of a milk duct and spreads through the wall into the surrounding tissue. The cancer becomes surrounded by scarlike material, which forms the lump that is detected.

Infiltrating Lobular Carcinoma

This type of cancer accounts for 5 to 10 percent of cases. Here the cancer starts in the cells lining the lobules and spreads through the lobule walls to the surrounding tissue. The cancer typically forms fingerlike projections rather than a lump and may be more difficult to distinguish and diagnose than infiltrating ductal carcinoma.

Ductal Carcinoma In Situ (DCIS)

Combined with lobular carcinoma in situ (below), this type of cancer accounts for 15 to 20 percent of cases. It starts in the cells that line the duct walls but has not spread outside the ducts. However, it may eventually involve a larger area of the ducts. If not treated, it may spread outside the ducts. It is the earliest stage of breast cancer.

Lobular Carcinoma In Situ (LCIS)

Combined with DCIS (above), this condition accounts for 15 to 20 percent of cases. LCIS originates in a lobular cell and grows within the lobule but has not spread to tissue outside the lobule. LCIS is considered a precancerous condition in which a premalignant change has occurred in the lobular cells. The cells divide and multiply but do not always become invasive cancer. Thus, LCIS is considered a marker for having an increased risk of developing invasive breast cancer in either breast.

Inflammatory Breast Cancer

This is the rarest form of breast cancer and accounts for 1 to 4 percent of cases. It invades and blocks lymph vessels in the skin, which results in a red, warm, swollen breast.

Diagnosis and Staging

If breast cancer is suspected and can't be definitively ruled out by a mammogram or ultrasound, a biopsy is performed to determine whether the cells are cancerous. The pathology report from the biopsy provides information about the size and type of tumor; whether it has spread into the blood vessels, lymphatic system, or surrounding fat tissue; its hormone receptor status; and other important characteristics. These findings, along with information obtained from other tests that may be performed, are used to stage the disease and determine the plan of treatment. Based on the size of the tumor and whether it has spread, breast cancer is assigned a stage from zero through IV, with Stage IV being the most severe. It is important to note that lymph nodes are not typically removed from under the armpit at the time of the biopsy. The removal and examination of these nodes (a procedure called axillary lymph node dissection) is performed at the time of breast surgery, if required.

Treatment and Side Effects

The treatment of breast cancer involves various combinations of four basic treatment options: surgery, radiation therapy, chemotherapy, and hormone therapy. The recommended course of treatment is determined by the results of the staging process and the individual characteristics of the patient. Each treatment option will be explored after a general discussion of side effects.

Side Effects

Many of the side effects of cancer treatment may affect your ability to exercise and your response to exercise. This is why *you must check with your doctor before you start.* She or he can help you understand your disease and treatment, the possible implications for your exercise program, and signs to watch for that may tell you to stop exercising.

Limited Mobility and Function

Among the side effects that can occur with surgery are tightness across the chest and stiffness in the arm and shoulder. These can result initially from the swelling caused by the surgery and then from the scar tissue that may form. These side effects can limit mobility and function and may cause pain with movement. If mobility is not restored, a condition known as frozen shoulder may occur. In this condition, inflammation and scar tissue form in the shoulder joint and make movement extremely painful and limited or impossible. It can take several months of intensive physical therapy to remedy this problem. Preventing the condition is easier than treating it. This is why initial range-of-motion and stretching exercises to restore function are vitally important to your recovery.

Postural Imbalance

Another possible side effect of surgery is back pain due to a postural imbalance created by the removal of one breast without reconstruction or prosthesis. In this situation, guarding of the area may become normal. This guarding can include rounding the shoulder forward, keeping the arm close to or across the body, limiting arm and shoulder movement, dropping the head forward, and rounding the back slightly forward to protect and hide the area where the breast was removed. All of these actions may alter the posture and result in stress on the back and tightening in the abdomen. The shoulder and neck muscles also may become tight and stiff because of limited movement and the forward, rounded position.

Lymphedema

Lymphedema is swelling produced by an accumulation of lymph fluid in tissue. For breast cancer patients, the swelling occurs in the arm on the affected side due to damage to the lymph vessels in the armpit area caused by the removal of lymph nodes there (axillary lymph node dissection) or from radiation to that area. Removal of the nodes and damage to the lymph vessels prevent the lymph fluid in the arm from draining properly, allowing it to accumulate in the tissue. In addition, this damage may result in pain and tightness in the area as the lymph vessels close up, tighten, and sometimes snap.

If lymphedema is not treated, the swelling, which can affect the entire arm and hand, can result in decreased arm function, decreased range of motion and function in the fingers, and numbness in the hand. Moving your arm and contracting your muscles—as you do during exercise—so that the muscles "squeeze" the lymphatic vessels and help move fluid through them may possibly help prevent this condition.

While lymphedema may not occur immediately after surgery, it can occur at any time during the rest of your life after breast cancer treatment. Taking proper precautions in caring for your affected arm can help prevent the development of serious lymphedema.

Older individuals and those with poor nutrition face an increased risk of lymphedema, as do individuals with infections. Guarding against infection is extremely important because your affected arm will be more susceptible to infection than your unaffected arm, and infection can cause increased swelling. Be careful not to cut or scratch yourself when shaving your armpit or working in the garden or kitchen. Avoid insect bites, burns, skin irritants (such as strong detergents), hangnails, and torn cuticles. If you do cut or scratch yourself, wash and clean the area with soap and water, use an antiseptic, cover the injury, and keep the area clean to prevent infection. Avoid tight clothing and jewelry that could cause swelling. Do not receive shots, have blood drawn, or have your blood pressure measured in the affected arm. Also, if you are overweight and experience arm swelling, losing some weight can help reduce the swelling by reducing the amount of fatty tissue, which retains fluid.

If you notice any signs of infection, contact your doctor immediately. These signs include swelling, fever, or skin that is red, tender, warm, persistently itchy, or blotchy.

It is extremely important that you discuss lymphedema with your doctor or physical therapist (some physical therapists specialize in treating lymphedema). Ask questions and be sure you understand how to care for your arm, what signs to watch for, and what to do if you experience lymphedema. You can also contact the National Lymphedema Network (see the resources section) to get information and to find a lymphedema treatment clinic near you.

If you have lymphedema, you should not participate in the *Essential Exercises* program until you are cleared by your physician (and your physical therapist if you have one). You should also discuss using arm wraps with your doctor and physical therapist and strictly follow any instructions they give.

Potential Side Effects of Breast Cancer Treatment

PHYSIOLOGICAL EFFECTS

- Numbness in armpit and/or arm
- Pain in chest, upper back, and/or neck
- Loss of strength in chest and/or shoulder
- Loss of function in chest and/or shoulder
- Decreased overall level of fitness
- Decreased functional ability
- Postural weakness and/or deformity
- Weight gain
- Lymphedema

PSYCHOLOGICAL EFFECTS

- Loss of self-esteem
- Loss of identity
- Loss of sense of being in control
- Fear of intimacy or sexual dysfunction
- Fear of death
- Fear of disfigurement
- Fear of loss of independence
- Negative body image
- Depression

Aaronson (1997); Durak and Lilly (1997); MacVicar and Winningham (1986); MacVicar et al. (1989); Saccone (1995); Winningham (1991, 1992a, 1992b); Winningham and MacVicar (1988); Winningham, MacVicar, and Burke (1986); Winningham, MacVicar, Bondoc et al. (1989); Miaskowski (1997); American College of Sports Medicine (1997, 1998, 2000); Brown (1997, 1998).

CHRONIC EFFECTS

- Osteoporosis
- Type II diabetes

- Damage to heart or lungs
- Damage to nerve cells

NUTRITIONAL PROBLEMS
- Nutritional imbalance
- Anorexia
- Diarrhea
- Vomiting
- Nausea

BLOOD CELL COUNT
- Reduced blood cell counts, which may lead to suppressed immune function, susceptibility to fever, infection, fatigue, bleeding, or weakness.

Aaronson (1997); Durak and Lilly (1997); MacVicar and Winningham (1986); MacVicar et al. (1989); Saccone (1995); Winningham (1991, 1992a, 1992b); Winningham and MacVicar (1988); Winningham, MacVicar, and Burke (1986); Winningham, MacVicar, Bondoc et al. (1989); Miaskowski (1997); American College of Sports Medicine (1997, 1998, 2000); Brown (1997, 1998).

Surgery

Surgery involves the removal of the tumor in an operation. The procedure may be breast-conserving, such as a lumpectomy or partial mastectomy, or it may involve removal of the entire breast. When appropriate, surgery also may include removal of some of the axillary lymph nodes.

Following is a review of each surgical procedure and its possible implications for exercise. The gray portion of each diagram indicates the area most likely involved in the surgery.

Axillary Lymph Node Dissection

PROCEDURE   This procedure is performed in conjunction with many cases of breast cancer surgery. Some of the axillary (armpit) lymph nodes are removed for examination by a pathologist to determine how likely it is that the cancer has spread outside the breast. The surgeon can never be sure exactly how many nodes he or she is removing, because a mass of tissue containing the nodes is removed. Anatomically, there is an "axillary fat pad" and the number of nodes removed depends on how many nodes each individual has in that anatomical location.

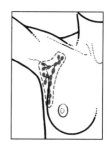

Axillary Lymph
Node Dissection

To remove the lymph nodes, the surgeon must remove the nodes from the lymph vessels to which they are attached. The higher into the armpit the surgeon goes, the more lymph nodes removed. This increases the trauma to the area. After the removal of the tissue and lymph nodes and the sewing back together of the skin, the underarm may have a deeper concave area and the skin may be tighter. Also, the lymph vessels that were severed in the procedure will close up and become tight.

IMPLICATIONS FOR EXERCISE   The tightness of both the skin and the closed-up lymph vessels can impair shoulder and arm function by making movement difficult and painful. Also, motor function in a shoulder girdle muscle, the serratus anterior, may be temporarily impaired and not work to stabilize the shoulder blade, causing feelings of weakness in the arm. The nerve that tells this muscle to function runs through the area of surgery, and the surgery may cause the nerve to cease firing temporarily. In the weeks after surgery, the nerve usually begins to come back to normal function, and the problem resolves itself. As sensory function returns, tingling, soreness, and burning may be felt along the upper inside of the arm and the outside of the chest wall.

Lymphedema is another potential side effect of axillary lymph node dissection. However, research has shown promising preliminary results for a new staging procedure known as sentinel node biopsy (discussed in the next section), which requires less invasive surgery and potentially reduces damage to the lymphatic system. As new techniques such as this are discovered and improved, the need to perform axillary lymph node dissection may be reduced.

If you have undergone axillary lymph node dissection, you should proceed slowly and cautiously in your exercise program. Begin with little or no weight and progress according to how your arm responds to the exercise. If you notice any signs of swelling, stop exercising and see your doctor. Always monitor your arm, and don't "work through" any achiness or heaviness. Also, have your doctor or physical therapist check for any possible nerve injury and muscular weakness. For more specific precautions, see "Points to Remember When Performing All Exercises" on page 46 and "At-Home Assessment Procedures" on page 40.

Sentinel Lymph Node Biopsy

PROCEDURE   This procedure is being studied as a means to identify women who are node-negative by identifying and examining what is called the sentinel lymph node. The sentinel node is the first node to receive lymph that drains from the cancerous area and will be the node most likely to contain cancerous cells if they have spread from the primary site. If this node is found to be clear of cancerous cells, it is thought that nodes beyond it also will be clear of disease. Sentinel node biopsy involves identifying the sentinel node by lymphatic mapping, a procedure in which the nodes that drain the tumor are identified. The sentinel node is then removed for examination by a pathologist.

IMPLICATIONS FOR EXERCISE   Unlike the painful and debilitating side effects that can occur with axillary lymph node dissection, this procedure results in a smaller scar in the armpit area and fewer painful complications. Women who are sentinel-node-negative may not need a full-scale axillary lymph node dissection. Because this is a relatively new procedure, there is not yet enough research available to definitively determine its accuracy. For a more detailed discussion of the procedure and its implications for exercise, ask your doctor and review the references in the resources and references sections.

With a sentinel node biopsy, you should still take care to begin your exercise program slowly and proceed cautiously, and ask your doctor when you can begin. Although the trauma to your lymphatic system is reduced, you must also take into account any other treatment that you have undergone.

Breast-conserving Surgery

PROCEDURE   Breast-conserving surgeries remove only the tumor and some of the normal surrounding breast tissue. These operations are often called lumpectomy or partial (also referred to as segmental mastectomy or quadrantectomy) mastectomy. Different surgeons may use different terminology. The amount of tissue removed is determined by the tumor's size and location in the breast. A goal of breast-conserving surgery is to remove enough tissue to include a "rim" of normal tissue all the way around the tumor. Surgeons call this a clear margin. As part of the procedure, lymph nodes may be removed to look for spread of the disease. Usually the lymph nodes are taken out through a separate incision. A three- to five-inch incision is made in the armpit area to remove the lymph nodes. Radiation treatment generally comes after breast-conserving surgery. Chemotherapy and hormone therapy also may follow.

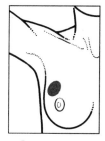
Lumpectomy

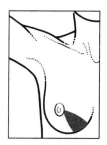
Partial
Mastectomy

IMPLICATIONS FOR EXERCISE   Use of this procedure may prevent some of the muscle weakness, infection, and lymphedema that can arise with more major surgeries. However, the axillary lymph node dissection and radiation therapy that accompany breast-conserving surgery may result in the same problems discussed previously. Like lymph node dissection, radiation can damage the lymphatic system and cause lymphedema and shoulder dysfunction. Radiation is discussed later in this chapter.

If you have undergone breast-conserving surgery, check with your doctor about when you can begin your exercise program. You should begin with range-of-motion exercises such as those in Level I (page 63) to make sure that you don't have any limitations in movement. Additional Level I exercises are also important to begin strengthening the muscles that stabilize your shoulder blades, allow for correct arm function, and preserve your upright posture.

Total (Simple) Mastectomy

PROCEDURE   This procedure involves total removal of the nipple-areolar complex, the breast mound, and possibly some skin, but no chest muscle is removed. Axillary lymph nodes usually are not removed, though nodes that are in the breast tissue are included in the tissue removed and examined. Radiation therapy may follow. This procedure is usually used for cases where the cancer is in situ or as a preventive measure for those at high risk to develop breast cancer (diagnosed with LCIS).

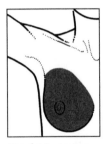

Total Mastectomy

IMPLICATIONS FOR EXERCISE   Skin tightness can result where the skin is sewn together on the chest after the breast is removed. In addition, skin can become "stuck" to the tissue below it (adhesions) as scar tissue forms. Scar tissue is thick, collagenous connective tissue laid down by the body in an attempt to repair injured tissue. In this case, the scar tissue is laid down in a pattern that prevents the normal "sliding of the skin" across the tissue below it. All of this can make movement painful and difficult.

Modified Radical Mastectomy

PROCEDURE   The nipple-areolar complex, the breast mound, the axillary lymph nodes, and the lining over the chest muscles are removed. In today's procedures, it is uncommon for muscles to be removed. Radiation may follow, depending on the size of the tumor, the number of lymph nodes included, and the status of the surgical margins.

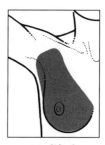

Modified
Radical
Mastectomy

IMPLICATIONS FOR EXERCISE   Modified radical mastectomy can result in muscular weakness, tightness of the skin over the chest area and in the armpit, tight and closed-up lymph vessels, adhesions of the skin to the chest muscle, and lymphedema. The main muscular problem is weakness of one of the shoulder girdle muscles, the serratus anterior, which can cause shoulder instability and limit certain shoulder movements. This weakness may be accentuated if there is injury to the pectoralis muscles or the nerves that stimulate them. The large chest muscle, pectoralis major, also may become tight and spastic. These complications can make it both difficult and painful to raise the arm.

Radical Mastectomy

PROCEDURE   This procedure is rarely performed today. Here the nipple-areolar complex, the breast mound, and some of the tissue around it are removed. Both chest muscles are removed, and an extensive axillary lymph node dissection is performed.

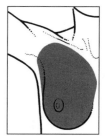

Radical
Mastectomy

IMPLICATIONS FOR EXERCISE   This aggressive procedure leaves a large depression on the chest wall. It can result in lymphedema, weakness in the arm muscles, arm numbness and discomfort, and limited shoulder motion.

Potential Side Effects of Surgery

MUSCULAR WEAKNESS

- Radical mastectomy (rarely performed) may result in weakness in muscles used for bringing the arm across the chest in a raised position (parallel to the floor) on involved side; weakness or decreased function of affected arm when large chest muscle (pectoralis major) is removed

- Radical mastectomy and modified radical mastectomy may result in trauma to long thoracic nerve due to lymph node dissection; may result in weakness of one of the shoulder girdle muscles (serratus anterior) and cause reduced shoulder stabilization and ability to rotate

the shoulder blade upward, limiting the ability to raise the arm out away
from the body and straight out in front of the body

- Postural weakness and/or deformity

CHEST WALL ADHESIONS
- Scar tissue formation on tissue lining chest wall after surgery; may result
  in decreased range of motion and function in arm or shoulder of
  affected side; may result in postural deformity of trunk

- Possible pulmonary problems

LYMPHEDEMA
- Removal of lymph nodes alters normal lymph circulation; results in
  swelling of affected arm

- Extravascular and extracellular fluids may gather in the tissue of the
  affected arm and result in swelling, increased size, and decreased function of arm; decreased range of motion in fingers; stiffness in fingers;
  and disruption of sensory function in hand

- May occur at any time

PAIN
- Pain in back of neck and shoulder area and muscle spasms due to guarding of muscles in those regions; tingling, soreness, burning along upper
  inside of arm and outside of chest wall

- Sore muscles that are tender to the touch (levator scapulae, infraspinatus, and teres major or minor); may inhibit active movement of
  shoulder

- Frozen shoulder due to reduced use or movement of affected arm; may
  increase chance of lymphedema

Radiation Therapy

PROCEDURE   Radiation uses high-dose X rays to shrink tumors and kill cancerous cells that may have been left behind after spreading away from a
tumor that was removed by surgery. You may hear these remaining cells
referred to as hidden cells, because they are not detected at the time of
surgery.

Radiation therapy can be administered internally through thin plastic tubes inserted into the affected area or externally through the use of specialized equipment. It is a local therapy, meaning that it is administered only to the affected area. The radiation kills cells by permanently damaging their DNA in a way that causes them to lose their ability to function and then die. Radiation is almost always used after breast-conserving surgery and may be used after mastectomy (see page 20) and in conjunction with other therapies in cases of advanced cancer. In cases where the cancer has spread to other areas of the body, radiation may be used to treat those areas.

IMPLICATIONS FOR EXERCISE Although everyone responds differently, most people experience few, if any, side effects. The most common are fatigue and skin effects. Some of the general side effects that can occur from radiation in other parts of the body—nausea, vomiting, hair loss—do not occur when radiation is limited to the breast. However, if the axillary lymph nodes also receive radiation, this can cause the lymph vessels to contract and shrivel up. This increases the likelihood of lymphedema in a lymphatic system that has already been damaged by axillary lymph node dissection. Mobility also may be affected by the tightening of the skin that can occur with radiation.

Although treatment procedures have improved, some serious side effects can occur with radiation. These side effects are less common than those mentioned previously and should be discussed with your doctor. They include damage to the ribs, which increases the risk of rib fractures; inflammation of the heart or lungs; nerve damage; and secondary cancers. Should you experience or suspect any of these side effects, work with your doctor to determine when and if an exercise program is appropriate for you. For more information on these conditions, contact a cancer organization such as the Cancer Information Service (see National Cancer Institute in resources).

Potential Side Effects of Radiation Therapy

- Fatigue
- Temporary burns
- Shoulder dysfunction
- Breast swelling
- Tightening of the skin
- Red, dry, or irritated skin
- Hardening of the surgical scar (fibrosis)
- Reduced white blood cell count
- Scarring of the heart or lungs (very uncommon)

- Breast tenderness, which may remain indefinitely
- Pain from inflamed chest muscles and nerves
- Acute inflammation of lung tissue, impairing oxygen transfer
- Death of fat tissue in breast, resulting in inability to lactate
- Scar tissue formation in axilla (armpit), which may inhibit flow of lymph through lymphatic system and result in lymphedema

Chemotherapy

PROCEDURE   Chemotherapy uses drugs to kill any cancerous cells that have traveled outside the breast. It may also be used to shrink tumors, either to reduce pain or to make surgery easier. Chemotherapy is a systemic treatment because it travels through the bloodstream and can kill cancer cells anywhere in the body. It is generally used in addition to surgery and radiation and is termed adjuvant therapy. If given before surgery, it is called neoadjuvant. After surgery and radiation, chemotherapy is used to kill any undetected cells that might remain in the body. Chemotherapy kills cancer cells by interfering with cell growth and division.

IMPLICATIONS FOR EXERCISE   Many chemotherapy drugs are used separately and in combination in breast cancer treatment. Each drug has its own side effects. As with radiation, people respond to treatment differently. Following is a list of the main chemotherapy side effects. Though rare, some long-term side effects of chemotherapy include heart damage, leukemia, and fertility problems. For more details on these side effects and their likelihood of occurrence, talk with your doctor or contact a cancer organization such as the Cancer Information Service (see National Cancer Institute in resources).

Potential Side Effects of Chemotherapy

- Hair loss, dry skin, or rash
- Weight gain
- Nausea, vomiting, or diarrhea
- Decreased appetite
- Damage to the circulatory system and heart muscle (cardiomyopathy or accelerated atherosclerosis)
- Nerve damage causing arm or leg tingling and numbness
- Muscular weakness
- Decreased blood cell counts, which may result in anemia, infection, or clotting problems

Hormone Therapy

PROCEDURE   Like chemotherapy, hormone therapy is a systemic adjuvant therapy designed to stop the growth of cancerous cells. In some cases of advanced cancers, hormone therapy alone is used as a primary therapy. Deciding how effective hormone therapy is likely to be is based on whether the cancer cells have estrogen and progesterone receptors, a woman's menopausal status, and whether the tumor is slow- or fast-growing. Having receptors (places on the surface of cells where the hormones can attach and thus signal the cells to grow and divide), being postmenopausal, and having a slow-growing tumor all indicate a better response to hormone therapy. Hormone therapy inhibits the growth of cancer cells by blocking the effect of estrogen on these cells. Hormone therapy also can involve surgery to remove the hormone-producing organs.

The most commonly used drug is tamoxifen (Nolvadex). It is important to note that hormone therapy for breast cancer is not the same as hormone replacement therapy taken by some women after menopause. Different drugs are used for the two therapies.

IMPLICATIONS FOR EXERCISE   Hormone therapy is easier to give and has fewer side effects than chemotherapy. Typically, hormone therapy results in the menopausal symptoms listed below. Though rare, other side effects include nausea, rash, blurred vision, blood clots, mood changes, and weight gain. For more details on these side effects and their likelihood, talk with your doctor or contact a cancer organization such as the Cancer Information Service (see National Cancer Institute in resources).

Potential Side Effects of Hormone Therapy

- Weight gain
- Hot flashes
- Sweats
- Irregular menses
- Vaginal dryness or irritation

Reconstruction

After mastectomy, several procedures exist for the reconstruction of the breast either at the time of surgery or at a later date. These procedures involve different degrees of invasiveness, recovery time, and rehabilitation needs, and each presents possible side effects that may affect mobility in the arm and shoulder. Additional side effects include muscular tightness, weakness, and spasms. Strengthening the back and abdominal regions is important for improving posture and relieving pain after reconstruction.

A brief overview of some of the problems associated with reconstruction is provided here. For more details on the specifics of these procedures, consult your doctor, support group, or a cancer organization such as the Cancer Information Service (see National Cancer Institute in resources).

Saline Implants and Tissue Expanders

PROCEDURE   A saline implant is a "balloon" filled with saline and placed beneath the skin either on top of or underneath the chest muscle. A tissue expander is similar but is only partially filled before placement. It too goes beneath the skin, either on top of or underneath the chest muscle, initially to stretch the skin. Then, at various times in the next few weeks, the surgeon fills the expander with more fluid. This process of "fill and stretch" is repeated until the expander is full.

IMPLICATIONS FOR EXERCISE   With these procedures, the main complication is capsular contracture, a condition in which scar tissue around the implant or expander hardens and then contracts. This can cause deformity, pain, and abnormal firmness in the breast. It occurs most often with implants that are placed underneath the chest muscle. Additionally, the large chest muscle (pectoralis major), which may be separated from the chest wall to create a "pocket" for the expander, may react by going into painful spasms. Relaxation, stretching, and isometric exercises can help relieve the pain.

Latissimus Dorsi Flap

PROCEDURE   In this procedure, a back muscle called the latissimus dorsi and a football-shaped area of skin from the back are brought to the front of the chest. This is done by creating a "tunnel" under the skin of the armpit and pulling the muscle through the tunnel and out the mastectomy scar in the front. The muscle is then used to form a breast mound or, more commonly, is folded to create a pocket in which an implant is placed. The skin taken from the back is sewn into place on the front of the chest with all the blood vessels remaining intact.

IMPLICATIONS FOR EXERCISE   In this procedure, the transfer of the back muscle to the chest to create the breast mound results in some weakness around the shoulder blade. However, other muscles that move the shoulder blade are able to take over for the transferred muscle. Other complications include tissue death, blood clots, infection, and longer healing time than after an implant procedure or no reconstruction at all.

Transverse Rectus Abdominis Myocutaneous (TRAM) Flap

PROCEDURE   In this procedure, a football-shaped section of skin, fat, blood vessels, and muscle from the abdominal area is pulled up through a "tunnel" under the skin of the upper abdomen to form a breast mound on the chest. The skin is sewn into place with all the nerves and blood vessels remaining intact.

IMPLICATIONS FOR EXERCISE   With the cutting and moving of one or both sides of the abdominal muscle, known as the rectus abdominis, weakness can occur in the abdominal area. This can produce back pain, hernia, and decreased trunk stability. The procedure can make standing up straight difficult because of the incision across the abdomen. All of this can negatively impact posture and create muscular stress and tension. You will need to stretch your abdomen, strengthen your back, and work on improving your posture. Other complications include tissue death, blood clots, infection, and longer healing time than after implants or no reconstruction.

Free Flap

PROCEDURE   This procedure is similar to the TRAM flap in that skin, muscle, fat, and blood vessels are transferred from the abdomen to the chest to make a breast mound. However, the difference is that instead of leaving all the tissue intact and tunneling it under the skin up to the chest, the tissue—blood vessels and all—is cut out and then reattached to the chest. This is much more complicated and intense surgery, as each tiny blood vessel must be reattached to ensure proper blood supply to the tissue. Tissue also may be taken from the thigh and the buttocks (gluteus maximus).

IMPLICATIONS FOR EXERCISE   Problems may include muscular weakness in the area from which the tissue was removed and stiffness and soreness where the tissue was reattached. Recovery time is longer than in other procedures because of the extensive nature of the surgery and the time needed for the reattached blood vessels to "take root." Other complications include flap, skin, or fat tissue death.

Nipple-Areolar Construction and Tattooing

PROCEDURE   A nipple and areola can be constructed out of skin from the breast mound or other area of the body. This is called a modified skate flap and is created during a second surgery, after the patient has finished with other treatment. The exact timing is determined by how quickly the patient heals from the original surgery. To achieve a natural pigmentation for the new nipple and areola, medical tattooing is performed.

PART II

Essential Exercises

CHAPTER 3

Getting Ready to Exercise

The exercise program encouraged me to practice my range-of-motion exercises. They also took my mind away from the discomfort I felt and the feeling of being no longer attractive. I was proud of myself and what I was able to do. I was energized.

Marlene Haffner, M.D., M.P.H.
Rear Admiral, U.S. Public Health Service

Things don't change, we do.   —*Henry David Thoreau*

ALTHOUGH YOU MAY be growing tired of hearing this, *it is essential that you have your doctor's permission before beginning this or any other exercise program.* You have been through intensive medical treatment, and it is imperative that you are physically and mentally ready to begin. Your physician's evaluation is critical for determining whether you are putting yourself at risk by exercising. Your doctor will assess your overall readiness based on how well you are healing, how you responded to treatment, and whether you have a condition that necessitates seeing a physical therapist.

It is for your own benefit, and the ultimate success of your recovery and rehabilitation, that you listen to the advice of your team of medical professionals. They can tell you exactly which muscles were affected by your particular surgery and how your treatment may affect your response to exercise. This information is especially important if you already have lymphedema.

General Information and Cautions

As stated in Chapter 1, the goals of this program are as follows:

- To enhance your energy level through physical activity
- To improve your posture by stretching tight muscles and strengthening weak ones
- To increase your range of motion through stretching and movement exercises (with an emphasis on the upper body)
- To strengthen the body's core stabilizers—the abdominal and lower back muscles—through targeted exercises and dynamic movement
- To improve your quality of life by enhancing your physical and mental condition through exercise training

The program focuses on improving range of motion and upper body strength as follows:

Range of Motion

- Shoulder flexion: raising your arm directly in front of you and overhead

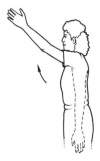

- Shoulder extension: pushing your arm straight back and behind you

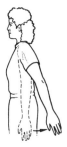

- Shoulder abduction: raising your arm straight out to the side

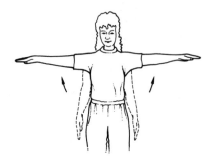

- Shoulder adduction: bringing your arm back to your side

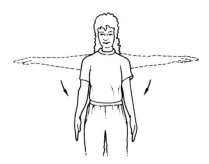

- Shoulder internal rotation: motion with your arm that causes the top of your arm bone (the "ball" of the arm bone that makes part of the shoulder joint) to rotate inward (toward your body)

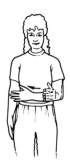

- Shoulder external rotation: motion with your arm that causes the top of your arm bone to rotate outward (away from your body)

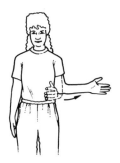

Upper Body Strength

- Chest muscles: pectoralis major and minor
- Back muscles: latissimus dorsi
- Shoulder muscle: deltoid

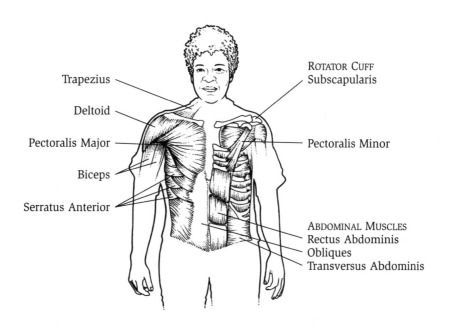

Trapezius
Deltoid
Pectoralis Major
Biceps
Serratus Anterior

ROTATOR CUFF
Subscapularis
Pectoralis Minor

ABDOMINAL MUSCLES
Rectus Abdominis
Obliques
Transversus Abdominis

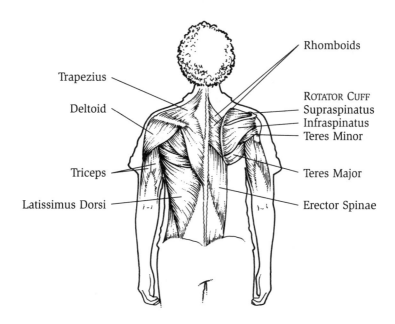

Trapezius
Deltoid
Triceps
Latissimus Dorsi

Rhomboids

ROTATOR CUFF
Supraspinatus
Infraspinatus
Teres Minor

Teres Major
Erector Spinae

- Shoulder joint stabilizers: rotator cuff muscles
- Back and shoulder girdle muscles: serratus anterior, middle and lower trapezius

Remember that this program is designed for those who are at least six weeks postoperative. When beginning, be aware of the symptoms and conditions listed on page 35. If any of them is present, you should not begin exercising. If any occurs while you are exercising, stop immediately. In either case, contact your doctor.

If you have undergone or are currently undergoing either chemotherapy or radiation therapy, you will have lower endurance and experience more fatigue. Moreover, your body may not be able to benefit fully from your exercise training, because treatments to destroy or slow the growth of tumors may hinder the body's ability to build protein. Even so, some benefit is better than none, and exercise should remain part of your rehabilitation program.

The side effects associated with chemotherapy and radiation, particularly fatigue and nausea, may make it difficult for you to follow a consistent training program and may lead to nutrition problems. You may experience a reduction in white blood cells, red blood cells, and platelets, increasing your risk of infection, anemia, and bleeding, respectively. However, it is important for you to remember that whereas one person may experience serious side effects with a type of treatment, another person may not. Thus, you may respond well to your treatment and may be able to exercise with few limitations.

If you are undergoing chemotherapy, it is important that you not let yourself get exhausted. Some days you may become nauseous or dizzy following your chemotherapy treatment. On those days, you may want to refrain from exercising or consult your physician before you do. It is suggested that you not perform any vigorous activity on days that you receive intravenous chemotherapy.

Likewise, avoid vigorous activity on days that you have lab tests done. Such activity can make test interpretation difficult and misleading. On days that you do not have lab tests or intravenous chemotherapy, try to perform some type of low- to moderate-intensity exercise. This can help decrease nausea and make you more aerobically fit at the end of your treatment.

Lymphedema has very important implications for exercise. In addition to observing the general caution about starting and progressing slowly, you must take extreme caution to protect your affected arm and watch for signs of swelling. Additionally, you must stress safety in your program—safety in

Warning Signs to Stop Exercising

Symptoms

- Chest pain or pressure
- Development of irregular pulse (irregular heart rate or palpitations)
- Development of resting pulse higher than 100 beats per minute
- Decreased heart rate or blood pressure during increased activity
- Excessive rise in blood pressure
- Recurring leg pain or cramps
- Sudden shortness of breath, muscular weakness, or tiredness
- Sudden onset of nausea
- Blurred vision, dizziness, faintness, or lightheadedness
- Vomiting or diarrhea within previous 24 to 36 hours
- Disorientation or confusion
- Pallor (paleness) or cyanosis (bluish skin)
- Fever

Treatment, Lab Values, or Blood Cell Counts (Obtained from Doctor)

- High-dose intravenous (IV) chemotherapy within previous 24 hours
- Platelet count below 50,000/mm^3
- Hemoglobin below 10 g/dl
- White blood cell count below 3,000/mm^3
- Absolute granulocyte count below 2,500/mm^3

Aaronson (1997); Durak and Lilly (1997); MacVicar and Winningham (1986); MacVicar et al. (1989); Saccone (1995); Winningham (1991, 1992a, 1992b); Winningham and MacVicar (1988); Winningham, MacVicar, and Burke (1986); Winningham, MacVicar, Bondoc et al. (1989); Miaskowski (1997); American College of Sports Medicine (1997, 1998, 2000); Brown (1997, 1998).

Here are some additional precautions you should observe.

- Reduce exercise intensity in response to very hot or humid environments or to altitudes above 5,000 feet.
- Avoid exercise when you experience tenderness in a joint that worsens with activity.
- Avoid strenuous aerobic activity during viral infections such as the flu or an upper respiratory tract infection.

exercise performance, equipment use, and environment. Perform exercises correctly and don't overdo it. Pay attention to the equipment and make sure you handle it safely and correctly. If you use an exercise band, use a towel or foam-covered handle to prevent putting too much pressure on your hand or other body part involved. The band should not be tight or restrictive. Also, don't let the band snap and hit you in your affected arm. If you use weights, handle them with care and make smooth and controlled motions. Also, if you work out with a friend or a group, watch out for your neighbors so that you don't bump into each other and thus risk injury. If you have lymphedema, avoid saunas and whirlpools and remember that tennis, golf, and racquetball are considered risky sports. If you have questions, locate a lymphedema specialist in your area.

Exercise in an environment that is clean, comfortable, and free of obstacles. Wear clothes that are loose-fitting, particularly on your arms, shoulders, and chest. You don't want to wear anything constricting, as it may be uncomfortable and may increase the risk of lymphedema. Make sure your clothes are appropriate for the climate in which you are exercising. Prevent yourself from overheating by wearing cool clothes and drinking plenty of water throughout your workout. Don't wait until you feel thirsty to drink; by that time, you are already getting dehydrated. Try not to eat a *heavy* meal within two hours of a workout. If you feel tired, listen to your body and either lower your exercise intensity or stop altogether. Getting plenty of rest and a good night's sleep also are essential parts of your exercise program.

Physical rehabilitation will be noticeably easier for those who were active prior to surgery. If you exercised before, there is no reason not to do so now. Just keep in mind that you cannot assume your previous training intensity immediately after surgery. You will have to build yourself back up slowly. Overtraining can result in impaired immune system function and fatigue.

If you were not active prior to surgery, your road to rehabilitation may be slightly longer. Start at a very low intensity and spend more time at each exercise level before progressing to the next.

Starting or restarting an exercise program after breast cancer treatment may feel a little like learning to walk again, but try not to get discouraged. Remember, you can do anything you were able to do prior to surgery, as long as you use a bit more caution at the start. When you exercise, you become physically and mentally stronger, which can help you cope with the challenges of breast cancer treatment. Exercise may be one of the best things you can do for yourself.

Flexibility

When we talk about flexibility, we are talking about your ability to move your joints through their full range of motion. You can assess your flexibility, which is specific to each joint and muscle group, by measuring your range of motion at a specific joint. You have probably seen a physical therapist with a protractor-like device called a goniometer, which is used to measure how many degrees you can move a joint. This measurement is referred to as your range of motion. Why is this important? It is important because a lack of flexibility can affect your ability to move normally and can increase your risk of injury and pain.

How flexible a person is depends on many factors, including the following:

- Age
- Gender
- Genetics
- Activity level
- Condition of connective tissue around joints
- Habitual posture
- Various diseases (osteoarthritis, rheumatoid arthritis, and any condition causing loss of mobility)

If you don't put each joint through its full range of motion, the muscles and connective tissue around it will respond by shortening. This makes movement difficult and sometimes painful. With regular stretching, you can improve your flexibility and range of motion.

The benefits of regular stretching include the following:

- Reduced muscle tension
- Increased range of motion
- Reduced risk of back injury and lower-back pain
- Good posture
- Greater awareness of body
- Possible reduction in risk of injuries
- General good feeling

Breast Cancer Treatment and Flexibility

Most relevant to your treatment for breast cancer will be your ability to move your shoulder joint through its full range of motion in all directions: flexion, extension, abduction, adduction, internal rotation, and external rotation (see definitions on pages 31–32). Also of concern is whether you have tightness and spasms in the muscles of your shoulder, chest, neck, and back. Your breast cancer treatment can both limit your movement and cause tightness and spasms, but these conditions can be improved by regular range-of-motion exercises—moving the joint as much as possible through its normal pattern of movement—and a regular stretching program.

After treatment and surgery for breast cancer, it's normal to feel tight, stiff, and sore in the muscles of the chest, back, shoulder, and neck. Your entire arm may feel this way and may be difficult to move. You also may have difficulty standing up straight. To help you begin your recovery and to prevent these symptoms from becoming worse, your physician may recommend that you begin physical therapy immediately following surgery to learn range-of-motion and stretching exercises. Although you probably won't feel like doing much of anything immediately after surgery, it's very important that you begin exercising at this time. If your doctor does not suggest physical therapy, be sure to tell him or her about difficulties you are having and ask for a referral to a physical therapist.

Range-of-motion and stretching exercises can help prevent frozen shoulder (see page 14). They are also an extremely important step in trying to prevent swelling and lymphedema. However, stretching is an important part of all exercise programs and should include the entire body. You will find a discussion on how to stretch in Chapter 4.

Weight Training

Flexibility is one of the five components of physical fitness. Of the other four—muscular strength, muscular endurance, body composition (fat-to-lean tissue ratio), and aerobic fitness—weight training will mainly help improve the first three.

With weight training, also called strength training, you won't tire as quickly and will feel stronger when doing physical work or recreational activities. Weight lifting also helps increase the amount of lean muscle in the body. Lean muscle burns more calories than fat when your body is at rest. This means you will burn more calories per day.

Weight training can help prevent or combat osteoporosis, a decrease in bone mineral density that can have crippling effects and can increase your risk of fracturing or breaking bones. Unfortunately, many women are sent into early menopause by breast cancer treatments, and this can increase the risk of osteoporosis. Weight training helps maintain or increase bone density and reduce or slow the effects of osteoporosis.

Weight training also offers psychological benefits. When you begin lifting weights, you are doing something challenging, and you will probably experience a significant increase in self-confidence and self-esteem as a result. Your body will look better, which will lead to a better self-image. These changes will carry over into other areas of your life.

The exercises in Chapter 4 provide some weight training benefits. For a more detailed discussion of weight training and its relationship to breast cancer treatment, see Chapter 6.

Monitoring Your Progress

If you go through physical therapy, your physical therapist will monitor your progress throughout your postsurgery range-of-motion and stretching program by measuring the range of motion in your affected arm and shoulder. After six weeks, enough healing should have taken place that you are ready to move to another level and begin your *Essential Exercises* program. The monitoring that takes place during physical therapy also will help determine the level of exercise best suited to your needs and physical condition when you make this transition. You will need to continue stretching those areas that are especially tight due to your treatment, but you should also begin including stretches for all the major muscle groups. *Essential Exercises* will walk you through this step-by-step. If you did not have physical therapy and have no formal record of your range of motion, you can begin now and track your progress throughout your program.

It's a great idea to keep a journal of how much and how often you exercise and what you eat. This gives you the opportunity to look back after a week or a month and determine how well you are sticking to your program. When tracking your exercise, include everything from walking the dog and gardening to more formal exercise activities. Record the amount of time spent on a particular exercise as well as the intensity at which you feel you worked, from very, very light to very, very hard (see page 185). You should probably never get to very, very hard; that intensity is too high for your purposes.

Record how you were feeling before, during, and after the exercise. If something hurts, make sure to write it down. It is important to discuss this pain with your doctor.

Measure the girth of your affected arm around your wrist, the largest part of your forearm, your elbow joint, and the middle of your upper arm both before and after exercise. Tracking these measurements allows you to watch for signs of swelling. Swelling, achiness, and a feeling of heaviness in the arm suggest that you are doing too much and trying to progress too fast. If you notice any changes in size or tissue texture of your arm, stop exercising and contact your doctor immediately. Remember, both the surgery and your post-surgery treatment take a great deal out of you, and the rehabilitation process will take time. Be patient with yourself; the results will come. Refer to "Points to Remember When Performing All Exercises" on page 46 for more on your measurements.

You can monitor your own progress in terms of range of motion by using the at-home assessment procedures in the next section.

At-Home Assessment Procedures

Before you begin your exercise program, take some initial assessment measurements to establish a baseline of information. Take these measurements again each month as you follow your program and record them on the sheet provided (see pages 42–43). This information will help you monitor your progress and decide when to advance to the next exercise level. Procedures for taking the various physical assessment measurements are outlined here. You may want a friend or family member to help you with some of the procedures. In some cases, you will need to see your doctor or a physical therapist before you continue.

You should see your doctor before you begin the assessment procedures if you have any of the following symptoms:

- Pain when moving your arms out to the side, up overhead in front of you, or behind you
- Feelings of muscular weakness when raising your arms in any direction or moving them behind you
- Extreme differences between arms in how far you can move them in various directions (forward, backward, up and out to the side, internal and external rotation)
- Any odd sensations that cause you concern or discomfort

At-Home Physical Assessment Sheet

Turn to the sheet beginning on page 42. Follow the procedures and record your results. When you reassess yourself, be sure to complete the sheet at the same time of day and before you have done any exercises.

Part A

1. Fill in the date, time of day, age, weight, and height blanks.

2. Calculate your body mass index (BMI) using this formula:
BMI = weight × (704.5/height²)
For example, for a woman who is 5 feet 4 inches (64 inches) tall and weighs 135 pounds, her BMI would be calculated as follows:
BMI = 135 × (704.5/64²)
= 135 × (704.5/4,096)
= 135 × .172 = 23.2
Use the chart below to determine your health classification in terms of your BMI.

BODY MASS INDEX	
	FEMALES AND MALES
Normal	18.5–24.9
Overweight (health risks begin here)	25.0–29.9
Grade 1 obesity	30.0–34.9
Grade 2 obesity	35.0–39.9
Grade 3 obesity (extreme obesity)	40.0 or higher

3. To measure your resting heart rate, or pulse, sit quietly for five to ten minutes. Then, using your wrist (radial artery) or neck (carotid artery), place the fingertips of your index and middle fingers (not your thumb) where you can feel your pulse. To take your wrist pulse, hold your hand with your palm up and find the groove just above the tendons and below the bone on the thumb side of your wrist, near your wrist fold. For your neck, place your fingers just under your jawbone and slide them down your neck in what feels like a natural groove. Your fingers should be just above and to the side of your voice box. Don't press too hard. Starting with zero, count your pulse for one minute and record the number of beats. Generally, the lower your resting heart rate, the

AT-HOME PHYSICAL ASSESSMENT SHEET

A.   Date: Time of Day: A.M./P.M.

Age: Weight: Height:

BMI [weight (lbs) × 704.5/height (in)^2]:   Classification:

Resting heart rate (beats per minute):

B.   SHOULDER RANGE-OF-MOTION MEASURES

COMBINED SHOULDER INTERNAL ROTATION AND EXTENSION

Putting my hand behind my lower back with
my palm facing away from my body, the back
of my hand reaches to:

___ the top of my buttocks*

___ the middle of my lower back

___ the bottom of my shoulder blade

___ the middle of my shoulder blade

___ the top of my shoulder blade

SHOULDER FLEXION

Raising my arms straight in front of me and up overhead (my palms are facing each other):

___   my arm is parallel to the ground (90° angle to the ground)*

___   my arm is slightly above my shoulder (120° angle to the ground)

___   my arm is pointing diagonally upward (150° angle to the ground)

___   my arm is pointing straight up to the ceiling (180° angle to the ground)

SHOULDER EXTENSION

Standing up straight and keeping my shoulders
down (no rounding or leaning forward), my
palms facing behind me, and my arms straight,
I can move my arms behind me:

___ just to behind my buttocks*

___ to a 45° angle from my buttocks

BILATERAL SHOULDER ROTATION AND ELBOW FLEXION

With one of my hands reaching behind my head (palm facing my body) and the other reaching
behind my back (palm facing away from my body), I can reach the:

TOP HAND (RIGHT)

___   back of my head*

___   base of my skull*

___   top of my shoulder blades

___   middle of my shoulder blades

___   fingers of top hand touch fingers
of bottom hand

BOTTOM HAND (LEFT)

___   top of my buttocks*

___   my lower back*

___   just above my lower back

___   bottom of my shoulder blades

___   fingers of bottom hand touch fingers
of top hand

TOP HAND (LEFT)	BOTTOM HAND (RIGHT)
___ back of my head*	___ top of my buttocks*
___ base of my skull*	___ my lower back*
___ top of my shoulder blades	___ just above my lower back
___ middle of my shoulder blades	___ bottom of my shoulder blades
___ fingers of top hand touch fingers of bottom hand	___ fingers of bottom hand touch fingers of top hand

C. SIMPLIFIED UPPER BODY POSTURAL ASSESSMENT

Asking a friend to help or using a full-length mirror, select the appropriate response or responses:

1. My head looks like it is   ___ jutting forward   ___ tilted right   ___ tilted left   ___ neutral.

2. My chin looks like it is   ___ tilted down   ___ level to the ground   ___ tilting up.

3. My shoulders look like   ___ they are rounded forward   ___ they are level   ___ the left is higher   ___ the right is higher.

4. When my arms are hanging at my sides, my palms ___ face (slightly or totally) behind me   ___ face my body   ___ face slightly forward.

5. My upper back looks   ___ rounded or hunched forward   ___ slightly curved   ___ excessively flat.

6. My shoulder blades look like they are   ___ flat and about 4 inches apart   ___ less than 4 inches apart   ___ more than 4 inches apart   ___ sticking out on bottom.

D. UPPER BODY ENDURANCE (WALL PUSH-UP TEST)

Date: Number of Wall Push-ups Completed:

E. ARM GIRTH MEASURES (INCHES)

Date: Side of body: Right/Left

Wrist fold (where wrist bends): _____   5 inches above wrist fold: _____

Elbow crease (where elbow bends): _____   5 inches above elbow crease: _____

F. SUBJECTIVE COMMENTS ON HOW I FEEL

1. I feel fatigued when I exercise.   ___ Yes   ___ No

2. I feel better when I exercise.   ___ Yes   ___ No

3. I feel energized when I exercise. ___ Yes   ___ No

4. Here are my thoughts on how I feel and how I am doing. (Use a separate sheet of paper.)

* May indicate that you have some limitations. However, some people are less flexible than others. If you are unsure of your condition, contact your doctor. If you have had a bilateral mastectomy and you fall into one of the asterisked categories, contact your physician for approval to begin your program or for referral to a physical therapist.

more fit you are. However, heart rate can vary for many reasons, so check with your doctor or an exercise specialist to learn more about your resting heart rate.

Part B: Shoulder Range-of-Motion Measures

To assess shoulder range of motion, follow the directions on the assessment sheet and check the appropriate response or responses as indicated. The movements should not be painful. You will use this information as your baseline and reassess yourself every month. If you find that you have severe limitations in movement on your affected side as compared to your unaffected side, consult your doctor immediately and do not begin the program until you get her or his approval. If you have had a bilateral mastectomy and you fall into one of the categories marked with an asterisk on the assessment sheet, contact your doctor for approval to begin your program or for a referral to a physical therapist. If you are unsure of your condition, consult your doctor.

Part C: Simplified Upper Body Postural Assessment

The purpose of the simplified upper body postural assessment is to look for certain postural imbalances that can result from your surgery or treatment. Postural imbalances also can result from many daily activities. It is important to identify them and make the proper corrections.

When you stand with good posture, you should find the following:

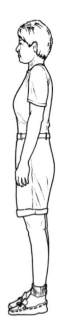

- Head: your head should be erect and centered, not jutting forward or tilted to either side.
- Chin: your chin should be level to the ground, not tilted up or down.
- Shoulders: your shoulders should be level, not rounded forward or one higher than the other.
- Palms: your arms should hang relaxed by your sides with your palms facing your body, not facing backward or forward.
- Upper back: your upper back should have a small curve to it, not exaggerated or hunchbacked in appearance or excessively flat.
- Shoulder blades: your shoulder blades should lie flat and be about four inches apart, not sticking out or too close or too far apart.

To perform your assessment, check the appropriate response or responses on the assessment sheet. If possible, have someone help you with this section. If you think you have postural imbalances, talk to your doctor to obtain a physical therapy consultation. A physical therapist can thoroughly evaluate your postural alignment and make the appropriate recommendations to correct any imbalances.

Part D: Upper Body Endurance

To assess your upper body endurance, follow the directions for the wall push-up on page 93. Record the number of wall push-ups you can do. You will use this number for comparison when you reassess yourself each month.

Part E: Arm Girth Measures (Inches)

Use a tape measure to measure the size of your arm at the points listed on the assessment sheet. You should also take your arm measurements before and after every exercise session. You can record these measurements in your personal exercise journal.

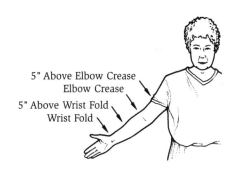

5" Above Elbow Crease
Elbow Crease
5" Above Wrist Fold
Wrist Fold

Part F: Subjective Comments on How I Feel

The last assessment item is extremely important. This is where you provide your subjective rating of how you are feeling and progressing in terms of your exercise. If you feel as if you are doing too much, slow down and progress at a slower pace.

Final Comments

For many of you, seeking the help of an exercise physiologist or certified exercise professional who is knowledgeable about breast cancer and its treatment may be an excellent way to begin your exercise program. These professionals will help you create a safe and effective exercise program, and they can provide emotional support and a bit of added persuasion. Whether you decide to do it on your own or with the assistance of a professional, you will be much more likely to stick with your program and remain injury-free if you start

Points to Remember When Performing All Exercises

- To begin strength training, you should be six weeks postsurgery and must have the permission of your physician.

- Make sure you warm up for five to ten minutes prior to performing any exercise. This can include five to ten minutes of easy walking or cycling and may include an additional five to ten minutes of stretching exercises.

- Do not hold your breath. Continue to breathe smoothly and consistently throughout your exercises. In general, exhale on exertion and inhale on the easier phase of an exercise.

- When performing an exercise, always move your arms in a slow and controlled manner; never drop them down carelessly.

- Progress slowly. Too many repetitions or too much weight can overwork muscles and may cause lymphedema. Don't work through sensations of achiness or heaviness.

- Progress at your own speed. Everyone is unique, and the amount of training you can do is very specific to you. Don't compare yourself to others.

- If you notice any redness, swelling, or heat in your affected arm, contact your physician immediately.

- Before you begin exercising, measure the girth of your affected arm around the wrist fold (where your wrist bends), five inches above the wrist fold, at the elbow crease (where your elbow bends), and five inches above the elbow crease. Take measurements after each exercise session to ensure that the affected arm does not swell to more than three-quarters of an inch greater than normal. In this way, you can monitor yourself for lymphedema. Also watch for swelling in your hands (across your knuckles), in the bony places in your arm (such as your wrist and funny bone), and in your armpit (axilla). If you notice any swelling, stop exercising and contact your doctor. It is important to catch any early signs of swelling and try to prevent it from becoming worse.

- Always warm up before and cool down after your exercise session—and always stretch when you are done.

slowly, progress slowly, and remain patient with yourself. And as we've stated before, *check with your doctor prior to beginning your exercise program.*

If you are interested in beginning this program but have not yet begun your treatment or are not six weeks postoperative, you can still use this book with your doctor's permission. If you are preoperative, you may want to do the at-home assessment (beginning on page 42), stretches (see page 51), and Exercises 10, 11, and 16 from Level I (see Chapter 4). If you are cleared by your doctor and want to do more or all of the Level I exercises, you can, but follow the principles for choosing exercises outlined on page 58. You may not have enough time before surgery to make big changes, but doing these exercises may help prepare you for exercising after surgery. The ideal situation would be to have a physical therapist evaluate your range of motion prior to surgery, but the at-home assessment will give you baseline measurements that you can compare to your postsurgery range of motion, determined by doing the assessment again after surgery.

If you are not six weeks postoperative, ask your doctor which Level I range-of-motion exercises you might be able to begin. You should, of course, be receiving guidance from your health care team regarding activities and movements that you can begin doing during the immediate postoperative period.

Whether you are just finished or long past your treatment, you can use this book. Get your doctor's approval, complete the at-home assessment, and begin slowly. Follow all the precautions discussed throughout the book, weigh any potential risks and benefits, and make your own decisions about exercise. Listen to your body and start on your own path to living stronger.

CHAPTER 4

The Exercise Program

[T]he program enabled me to surpass even my own expectations (which admittedly are quite high!). I am pleased to recommend it highly to any woman who might find herself in my situation.

Margaret McKaig

True life is lived when small changes occur. —Leo Tolstoy

IF YOU TURNED straight to this chapter to begin exercising, you missed some important information. Before you do any of the exercises, you should, at the very least, do the following:

- Obtain permission to exercise from your doctor (and your physical therapist if you have one).
- Read the "Lymphedema" discussion on page 15.
- Review "Warning Signs to Stop Exercising" on page 35.
- Review "Points to Remember When Performing All Exercises" on page 46.
- Complete the "At-Home Physical Assessment Sheet" on pages 42–43.

You might also want to review the *Essential Exercises* program goals on pages 2–3 and the affirmations on page 8.

The best thing, of course, would be for you to read the first three chapters entirely. The information there will help you understand the relationship between your breast cancer treatment and your exercise program.

Program Overview

The exercises in this chapter are organized in five sections. The first section includes sixteen stretching exercises covering all of the body's major muscle groups. It is important that you include these stretches in every stage of your exercise program. The other four sections contain the flexibility and strengthening exercises that make up the *Essential Exercises* program. Each section, or level, contains more than twenty exercises, and each is more difficult than the one before.

Your exercise routine will consist of the following four components.

- General warm-up and prestretch
- *Essential Exercises* (Level I, II, III, or IV)
- Cooldown
- Flexibility exercises

General Warm-Up and Prestretch

As with any exercise program, you should begin your *Essential Exercises* program with a warm-up. The warm-up should include five to ten minutes of continuous rhythmical movements involving both the arms and the legs. For example, you could ride a stationary bike, walk outside or on a treadmill, or march in place. You should move your arms slowly and gently to prepare them for exercise. This can include moving them in the same patterns that you will be doing in your exercise segment. Be cautious in warming up your arms; don't begin the activity too quickly or in an uncontrolled manner. You must not overload your affected arm with a sudden rush of blood. The purpose of the warm-up is to increase circulation and body temperature and prepare your body for exercise.

At the end of your five- to ten-minute warm-up, you should do a prestretch of the major muscle groups. (The *Essential Exercises* program also contains a separate stretching component to be performed after your cooldown, when your muscles are warmest and most pliable. See "Flexibility Exercises" later in this chapter.)

Essential Exercises (Levels I, II, III, and IV)

These exercises are designed to improve range of motion and flexibility in the shoulder and chest areas, to restore strength to the shoulder and arm muscles, and to "train" the affected side to better handle the flow of lymph. Regardless of your personal exercise history, start with the Level I exercises and advance slowly and cautiously.

You will need to understand three terms to perform the exercises properly: repetitions, sets, and resistance. A *repetition*, or *rep*, is one performance of an exercise, from the starting position through the required movement pattern and back to the starting position. A *set* is made up of a certain number of repetitions. *Resistance* is added to make an exercise more difficult. Weights and an exercise band are forms of resistance.

At each level of your exercise program, you will begin with one set of 8–12 repetitions of each exercise. Please note that when you are beginning, do only what is comfortable for you. If you need to start with fewer than 8 repetitions, do so. The most important thing is to begin slowly. As you continue with your program, you will progress to performing two or three sets of each exercise. Some of the exercises can be done with weights, an exercise band, or a dowel, but this equipment is usually optional, especially in the lower levels.

Remember, your affected arm's response to exercise is your ultimate indicator for progressing to more reps, more sets, or the next level. If you feel pain or notice redness, change in skin texture, or swelling, stop exercising and call your doctor immediately. After you get permission from your doctor to begin exercising again, reduce the number of repetitions you do and the resistance you use (if any). Again, your arm's response will be your barometer.

Cooldown

After you have completed your exercise session, cool down for five to ten minutes. A cooldown includes slowing down your movements—without completely stopping—to let your heart slow down. You may do the same movements that you did in your warm-up, only at a slower and slower pace. The idea is to return your body to its pre-exercise state and to prevent blood from pooling in your arms and legs. After the cooldown, you will move into the final component of your exercise routine: a series of stretches for all the major muscle groups.

Flexibility Exercises

Flexibility, or stretching, exercises should be performed for all the major muscle groups: chest, back, shoulders, arms, and legs. As a breast cancer survivor, you want to focus on stretching your neck, chest, armpit, shoulder, and arms. Sample stretches are found in the next section; these are designed to address the specific concerns of breast cancer survivors. You should do additional stretching of those areas involved in your breast cancer treatment that may be especially tight; some of the chest and shoulder range-of-motion exercises in Level I work well here.

Stretching Exercises

Follow these recommendations.

- Always begin with a 5- to 10-minute warm-up.
- Never stretch to the point of pain, and don't lock your joints.
- Inhale as you begin each stretch. As your body eases into the stretch, exhale and try to stretch a little farther. Hold each stretch for 15–30 seconds.
- Repeat each stretch 1–3 times.

This component of your exercise program can be done both before and after the exercises. But if you are going to stretch only once (not suggested), do it after you have completed all of your exercises and your cooldown. Always warm up for at least 5 minutes prior to stretching (even if you are only going to stretch). You don't want to stretch a cold muscle.

Chest One

Stand with your feet shoulder width apart, facing a corner where two walls meet. Lift your arms gently toward the ceiling and place one arm on each wall. Bend both elbows, creating a 90-degree angle. Lean forward just enough to feel a mild pulling sensation across your chest. (If you don't have a corner, you can perform this stretch in a doorway. Stand just outside the doorway with your feet shoulder width apart. Lift your arms gently toward the ceiling. Place a forearm against each side of the door. Lean forward until you feel a good stretch across your chest.)

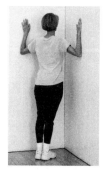

Chest Two

Stand an upper arm's length away from the wall, with your affected side toward the wall. Raise your arm so that the upper arm is in line with your shoulder or slightly below, your elbow is bent at 90 degrees, and your forearm is perpendicular to the ground (fingertips point straight up toward the ceiling). Place your forearm on the wall with your palm flat. Keeping your forearm and palm flat against the wall, gently turn your body away from the wall. Repeat on the other side.

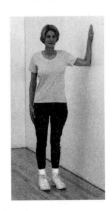

Upper Back One

Stand with your feet shoulder width apart. Clasp both hands in front of your body and raise your arms so they are parallel to the ground. Round your shoulders and gently pull your arms forward, away from your body, until you feel a mild stretch across your upper back.

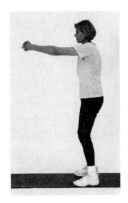

Upper Back Two

Find a well-grounded object such as a treadmill or post. This object should not move when you pull on it. Place one hand on the object and stand with your feet shoulder width apart facing the object. Round your shoulders and gently lean back, letting your body weight stretch your upper back and sides of your back. Your other arm will hang at your side. Relax to get the full benefit of the stretch. Make sure you don't lock your knees. Repeat with the other arm.

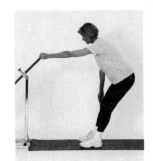

Lower Back One

Lie on your back with your knees bent and your feet flat on the floor. Put your arms around both legs and gently pull them in toward your chest. Be sure to grab your legs around the back of the thighs so that your lower legs are "on top of" your arms. Don't grab the tops of your lower legs and pull them into your body in such a way that you put a lot of pressure on your knees. Go only as far as is comfortable. This is a very subtle stretch, and it will not be obvious which muscles you are stretching.

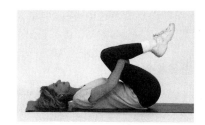

Lower Back Two

Position yourself on all fours. Round your back and press it up toward the ceiling like a cat. Relax to a flat-back position. After repeating 3 times, keep your hands in the same position and sit all the way back on your heels. Walk your fingers out in front of you as far as they will go.

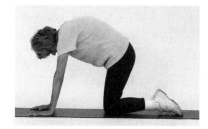

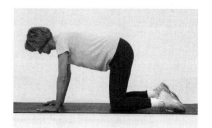

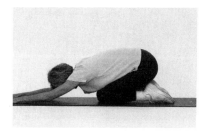

Neck One

Standing upright, look straight ahead with your chin level to the ground and your shoulders down and relaxed. Walk your left hand over your head and place it on your right ear. Gently pull your head over toward your left shoulder. Let your right arm hang at your side. (To help you hold your shoulder down, you can place your right arm behind your back with your elbow bent at a 90-degree angle.) Repeat on the other side.

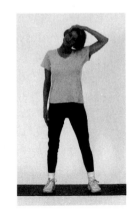

Neck Two

Standing upright, look straight ahead with your chin level to the ground and your shoulders down and relaxed. Tuck your chin and gently press your chin down to your chest. Hold the stretch and repeat.

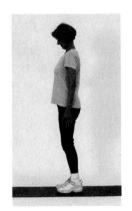

Shoulders One

Hold both arms out to your sides, keeping them parallel to the floor. Make large circles (of a size that is comfortable for you) with both arms in a slow and controlled manner. Be sure to go forward and backward, repeating 5–10 times in each direction.

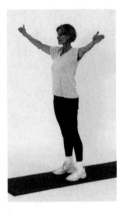

Shoulders Two

Standing upright, look straight ahead with your chin level to the ground and your shoulders down and relaxed. Bend one arm at the elbow and place the hand over the opposite shoulder. Take the other hand and gently press the slightly bent elbow toward your body. Be sure to keep your shoulders down as you press your arm toward your body.

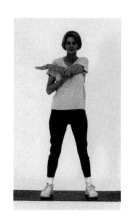

Biceps

Stand with your feet shoulder width apart, facing a wall. Extend one arm in front of you, with the palm of your hand flat against the wall. For the right arm turn counterclockwise, and for the left arm turn clockwise, until you feel the stretch through your upper arm.

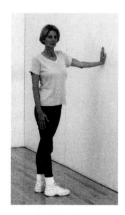

This exercise can also be performed by standing an arm's length from a wall with your palm on the wall and your fingers pointing behind you. To feel the stretch in your biceps, gently turn away from the wall while keeping your palm flat on the wall. You may feel the stretch all the way down your arm to your fingers as well as in your biceps.

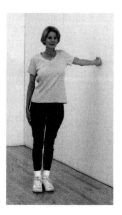

Triceps

Standing upright, look straight ahead with your chin level to the ground and your shoulders down and relaxed. Extend one arm over your head, letting it bend at the elbow so that your hand and forearm are behind your head. Grasp that elbow with the opposite hand and gently pull it toward the opposite side of your body. This stretch may be a bit more difficult on the side of the affected arm. Use your judgment; if it's too painful, skip this stretch and try it another day.

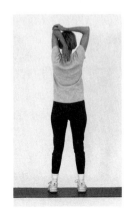

Quadriceps

Stand with your right hand against a wall or hold on to a chair for support. Bend your left leg and grasp your ankle with your left hand. Do not pull your heel into your buttocks as this can put too much pressure on your bent knee. Keep your back straight and your pelvis forward. Keep your knee under your hip. To get the most effective stretch, keep your foot flexed rather than pointed. Repeat on the right side.

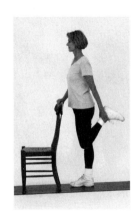

Hamstrings

Lie on your back with both legs extended in front of you. Bend one knee so that your foot is flat on the floor. Raise the other leg, knee slightly bent, and clasp both hands behind your thigh. Keeping the knee slightly bent, gently pull your leg toward your body. Don't let your buttocks come up off the floor. For more of a challenge, straighten your bent knee (the leg on the floor) and do not allow it to lift up off the floor as you pull your other leg toward you. Switch legs and repeat.

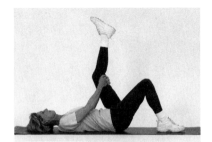

Buttocks

Lie on your back with both legs bent and your feet flat on the floor. Cross your left leg over your right leg so that the part of your lower leg above your left ankle rests on your right thigh. With or without the assistance of your hands, gently pull the right knee toward your body by clasping your hands behind your right thigh. Keep your head and neck on the floor and keep your shoulders relaxed (no hunching them up around your ears). You should feel the stretch across your left hip and buttock. Repeat with the other leg.

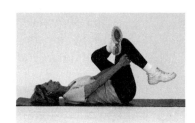

Calf

Stand with your feet shoulder width apart, facing a wall. Place both hands on the wall. Bend your right knee while extending your left leg behind you to the point where you are barely able to touch your heel to the floor. Press your heel to the floor and hold it there. You will feel the stretch in the lower part of your leg. Repeat on the right side. Perform the same exercise but this time bend your back knee. You should feel a slightly different stretch.

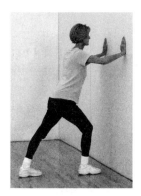

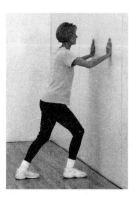

Range-of-Motion and Strengthening Exercises

You should perform range-of-motion exercises every day for the first year. Begin the strength training program when you are at least six weeks past your surgery and have your doctor's permission. Everyone should start with Level I. This level focuses mainly on range of motion, flexibility, and teaching you the movements for some of the more difficult strength exercises. You will be strengthening your postural muscles and shoulder girdle stabilizers (muscles that move, stabilize, and hold your shoulder blades and collarbones in the right place), but you will be using little, if any, resistance. If you pass the self-assessment at this level, you can move on to Level II (with your doctor's permission).

Level II is the beginning of the strength training program. When we refer to strength training, we are speaking only about the exercises in levels II, III, and IV of this book. We are not referring to any other program (even though others could apply). Any exercise in which an outside "load" is placed on the muscle is considered strength training.

As you progress through the *Essential Exercises* program, you will build strength and flexibility in your upper and lower body. Gradual, progressive stretching and strengthening of the arm, chest, shoulder, and back muscles will make you stronger, keep you fit, help improve your posture, and possibly help the flow of lymph fluid through your affected arm. It is reasonable for you to aim to do whatever you did before your surgery, as long as you don't have pain or noticeable swelling in your arm. It is important not to try to do too much too soon.

Do the exercises in the order in which they are presented. In this way, you will begin with the largest muscle groups and work your way to the smaller ones. It is important to adhere to this principle, as the larger muscle groups require more work (or heavier resistance) than the smaller ones, and if you tire the smaller ones first, you may not be able to complete (with good form) the exercises for the larger muscle groups. This also could put you at risk for injury.

If you can't complete all the exercises, do just a few. When choosing which exercises to do, remember to balance the muscle groups, work the groups that are important to you, and focus on your core stabilizers.

To balance muscle groups, pick exercises that work opposing muscles; that is, if you work the front of your upper arm, you should also work the back of your upper arm. This balancing can be done on the same day or over the course of a week, as long as, at the end of the week, you have given the same amount of work to the opposing muscle groups. The only time this may not apply is when working the postural and stabilizer muscles in the upper back. It is OK to work those muscles a little more than the opposing chest muscles, which tend to be tight and overworked anyway compared to the back muscles.

Besides balancing muscle groups, pick exercises that address any concerns identified by your at-home assessment (see pages 42–43) or your health care team. Also, focus on your upper body core stabilizers, as strengthening these muscles is important to proper arm function and warding off injury. These muscles include your middle and lower trapezius, rhomboids, latissimus dorsi, rotator cuff, chest, and serratus anterior.

Another approach is to begin with just the first few exercises, in the order in which they appear, and add to them as you go. Apply the principle of balancing muscle groups when deciding where to stop. If you have questions, ask your doctor or physical therapist for guidance.

Remember, more is not better. Initially, you may have low endurance and be able to work out for only a few minutes. Exercising at the same time each day is a good idea for consistency and compliance. Be faithful to your exercise regimen; with some determination and persistence, you will see great improvement in a relatively short time. As you begin to feel more comfortable with your routine, gradually increase the intensity of your exercise. As long as there is no pain or swelling, use your arms as much as you can, but don't work through any achiness or feeling of heaviness.

Exercise Instructions

Each exercise has two names: a technical name based on the muscle and joint movements that make up the exercise and an "analogy" name. The analogy name—such as "Starting the Lawn Mower" or "Swan Dive"—describes the activity or image that the exercise mimics. These names help make the exercises easier to understand and relate to. In addition, connecting the exercises to everyday activities helps you see the importance of exercise in maintaining your independence and improving your quality of life.

The "Description of Exercise" section gives step-by-step instructions for each exercise and suggests how many repetitions and sets to try to perform. A photograph accompanying the description illustrates good technique. If you can't stretch as far or bend as low or repeat a movement as many times as the description calls for, do only as much as you can. Don't risk injury by forcing yourself. With time and practice, you will be able to do more.

If you choose to purchase equipment, you may want: a one-inch diameter dowel, sets of one- to five-pound dumbbells, one- to five-pound adjustable ankle weights, an exercise band (preferably with padded handles), and a fifty-five-centimeter rubber exercise ball.

Each exercise includes "Starting Position" information. A proper starting position provides you with a comfortable, well-balanced base for making smooth, even movements. This may help protect you from injury and enables you to get the full benefit from your exercise. A proper starting position also reinforces good posture, and regaining good posture after surgery is a goal of the *Essential Exercises* program.

Each exercise also includes a "Purpose," and most include "Main Muscles Worked." Some Level I exercises do not list muscles worked because the exercises focus on stretching and range of motion rather than strengthening.

The following pages contain detailed descriptions and photographs of the six starting positions used for most of the exercises in this book. The exercises themselves, starting with Level I, follow these descriptions.

Starting Positions

A   Stand up straight with your arms at your sides, your feet shoulder width apart, and your knees slightly bent. Contract your abdominals and lower back muscles (putting your pelvis in the "neutral position," which maintains the natural curve of your spine). Pull your shoulders down and back and lift your chest—but not so much that you arch backward. Look straight ahead.

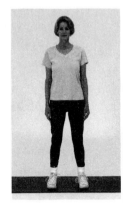

B Lie on your back on the floor, with your knees bent and your feet flat on the floor and hip width apart. Contract your abdominals and press the small of your back into the floor (pelvic tilt). Rest your arms straight at your sides with your palms down.

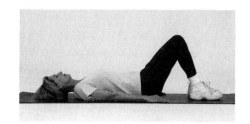

C Get on your hands and knees on the floor. Place your hands directly beneath your shoulders (fingers facing forward), your arms straight but not locked. Your knees should be shoulder width apart. Hold your head and neck in a neutral position (neither hanging down nor bent back), a natural extension of the spine.

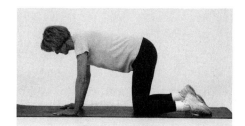

D Lie on your back on the floor, with your legs straight. Rest your arms straight at your sides with your palms down.

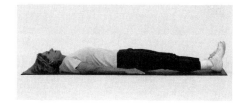

E Stand up straight with your hands on your hips, your feet wider than shoulder width apart, your toes turned out slightly to the side, and your knees slightly bent. Contract your abdominals and lower back muscles (putting your pelvis in the "neutral position," which maintains the natural curve of your spine). Pull your shoulders down and back and lift your chest. Look straight ahead.

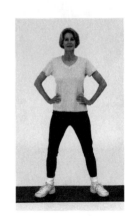

F Stand up straight with your arms at your sides, your feet together, and your knees slightly bent. Contract your abdominals and lower back muscles (putting your pelvis in the "neutral position," which maintains the natural curve of your spine). Pull your shoulders down and back and lift your chest—but not so much that you arch backward. Look straight ahead.

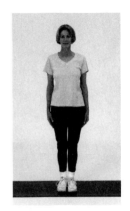

Level I

Level I consists of exercises specifically designed to improve range of motion and flexibility in the shoulder and chest areas, to begin conditioning the shoulder and arm muscles, and to start "training" the affected side to better handle the flow of lymph. Begin by building up to one set of 8–12 repetitions of each exercise. Some of you may progress to two to three sets of 8–12 repetitions of each exercise. Some of the exercises may include the use of 1- to 5-pound weights (stick with 1–2 pounds if you have not been exercising). Be sure to read all of the instructions under each exercise in Level I as some of the range-of-motion exercises include instructions on number of sets and repetitions that vary from the above instructions.

Remember that you do not have to exercise to the maximum position shown in the photograph or described in the text. Do only as much as you can. Remember also to move forward cautiously and always to monitor the arm on your affected side.

Advance to Level II only when you satisfy these conditions:

- You can perform either the number of sets and repetitions listed for each exercise, or two to three sets of 8–12 repetitions for all exercises in Level I.
- You have achieved range of motion on your affected side that is similar to your unaffected side.
- You have not experienced any negative responses in your affected arm (including swelling, achiness, numbness, redness, tissue texture change).
- You feel ready.

Continue to perform your Level I range-of-motion exercises even after you progress to the higher levels.

Take a minute to review "Points to Remember When Performing All Exercises" on page 46. Listen to your body and create your own plan for living stronger.

Level I Exercises

	TECHNICAL NAME	ANALOGY NAME
Exercise 1	Pendulum Exercise	Stirring Soup
Exercise 2	Butterfly	Butterfly
Exercise 3	Fingertip Wall Walk —Arm to the Side/Front	Raising Your Hand

Exercise 4	Head Walk	Monkeying Around
Exercise 5	Shoulder Extension	Swan Dive
Exercise 6	Pull Over	Good-Morning Stretch
Exercise 7	Side-to-Side Arm Push	Vaudeville
Exercise 8	Back Scratcher	Scratching Your Back
Exercise 9	Traffic Cop	Traffic Cop
Exercise 10	Corner or Wall Chest Stretch	Spying Through a Window
Exercise 11	Shoulder Blade Squeeze	Chicken Wings
Exercise 12	Arm Raise to the Front	Victory
Exercise 13	Arm Raise to the Side	Eagle Flapping Its Wings
Exercise 14	Biceps Curl	Popeye
Exercise 15	Arm Extension (Triceps)	Quarterback Throwing a Football
Exercise 16	Serratus Reach	Reaching for the Stars
Exercise 17	Lower Back (Floor Work)	Bridging
Exercise 18	Pelvic Tilt	Strong to the Core
Exercise 19	Abdominal Stretch	Lion
Exercise 20	Swami Stretch	Swami
Exercise 21	End-to-End Stretch	Elongation

Exercise 1: Pendulum Exercise

Stirring Soup

PURPOSE

To relax and loosen the arm and shoulder and to increase range of motion in the shoulder of the affected side.

STARTING POSITION A

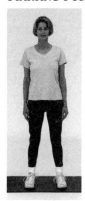

- Stand up straight
- Arms at your sides
- Feet shoulder width apart
- Knees slightly bent
- Abdominals contracted
- Lower back muscles contracted
- Shoulders down and back
- Chest lifted
- Look straight ahead

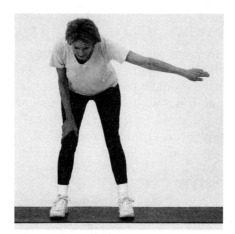

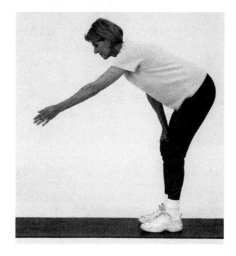

DESCRIPTION OF EXERCISE

1. Bend forward so that your chest is parallel to the floor. (If this is uncomfortable on your back, bend over only as far as is comfortable.) Rest your forearm (on your unaffected side) on a table, chair, or counter. If such a stationary object is not available, place your palm on your thigh on the same side, keeping your elbow slightly bent. Keep your abdominals contracted to protect your back. **2.** Slowly swing your affected arm from side to side (left to right) 8–12 times. **3.** Slowly swing the arm back and forth (head to leg) 8–12 times. **4.** Slowly swing the arm in a wide clockwise circle 8–12 times and then in a counterclockwise circle 8–12 times. **5.** Repeat with the other arm.

Be sure not to rest all of your body weight on the affected arm. Stop the exercise if you feel any pain or discomfort in the affected arm when it is used to support the position of your trunk.

You may choose to perform this sequence a second time. If you do, stand up straight in between the first and second sequence, raise your arms up over your head, and open and close your hands 5–10 times.

Steps 1–4 can be repeated throughout the day, particularly if you feel tense or tight in your arm and shoulder.

Level

I

Butterfly

PURPOSE

To loosen tight chest muscles and skin under the arm and to increase range of motion in the shoulder (external rotation). If you have shoulder problems such as tendinitis or bursitis, this exercise may be painful and should not be performed. The pain may be felt on the outside of the upper arm or on the corner of the shoulder.

STARTING POSITION A

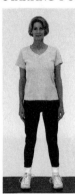

- Stand up straight
- Arms at your sides
- Feet shoulder width apart
- Knees slightly bent
- Abdominals contracted
- Lower back muscles contracted
- Shoulders down and back
- Chest lifted
- Look straight ahead

DESCRIPTION OF EXERCISE

1. Raise your affected arm to the side and put the palm of your hand on the back of your head or behind your ear. Keeping your shoulders down and your fingertips touching the back of your head or ear, move the elbow forward and back 8–12 times, like a butterfly flapping a wing. **2.** Repeat with the other arm. **3.** Raise both arms and put both palms behind your head or behind your ears. Move both elbows forward and back 8–12 times. Always move your arm(s) in a slow and controlled manner.

Perform steps 1–3, 1 time. This exercise can be done two or three times a day.

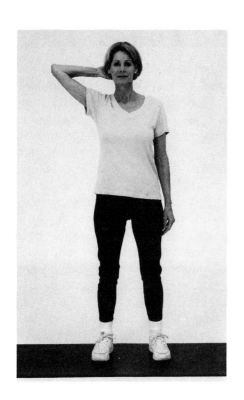

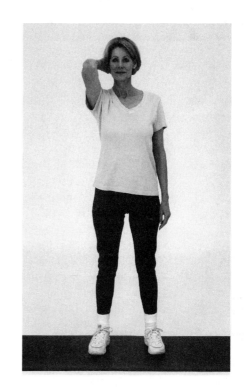

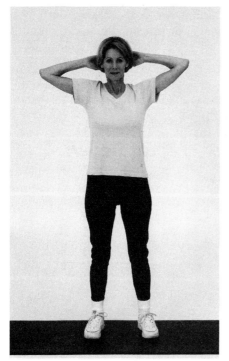

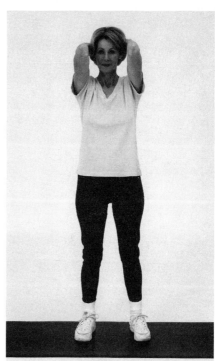

Exercise 3: Fingertip Wall Walk—Arm to the Side/Front

Raising Your Hand

PURPOSE

To increase range of motion in shoulder abduction.

STARTING POSITION A

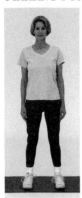

- Stand up straight
- Arms at your sides
- Feet shoulder width apart
- Knees slightly bent
- Abdominals contracted
- Lower back muscles contracted
- Shoulders down and back
- Chest lifted
- Look straight ahead

DESCRIPTION OF EXERCISE

1. Stand sideways an arm's length from the wall with your affected arm and shoulder toward the wall. **2.** Reach your arm out to the side and place your fingertips on the wall. "Walk" up the wall with your fingers as high as you can. Keep your shoulders down (no shrugging). Do not arch your back. You can bend your elbow slightly, but avoid leaning too much to the side. **3.** Return your hand to the starting position and repeat the motion 8–12 times. Each time, try to reach a little higher. It's normal to feel a slight pulling sensation in your muscles, but stop if you feel pain. **4.** Repeat with the other arm. **5.** Turn so that you face the wall and repeat steps 2 and 3 with your arms out in front of you. In this step you will do the exercise with both arms at the same time.

Perform steps 1–5, 1 time. You may move your feet in toward the wall if you need to as you reach higher with your arms.

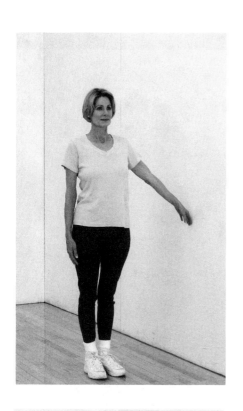

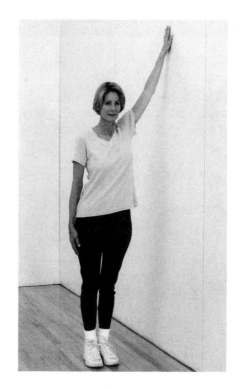

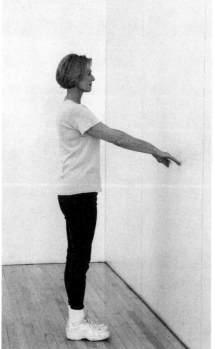

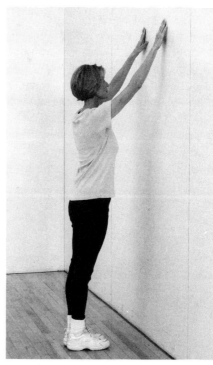

Exercise 4: Head Walk

Monkeying Around

PURPOSE

To stretch the shoulder, chest, axilla (armpit), and skin and to increase range of motion in the shoulder, armpit (axilla), and chest wall.

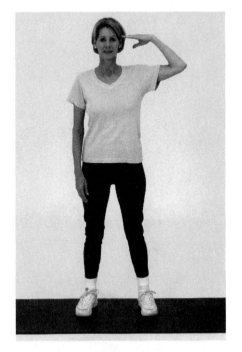

STARTING POSITION A

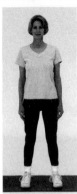

- Stand up straight
- Arms at your sides
- Feet shoulder width apart
- Knees slightly bent
- Abdominals contracted
- Lower back muscles contracted
- Shoulders down and back
- Chest lifted
- Look straight ahead

DESCRIPTION OF EXERCISE

1. Place the fingers on your affected side above your ear, with your elbow pointing out to the side. **2.** Walk your fingers across the top of your head to the other ear. Keep your elbow pointing out to the side. Keep your head straight—don't lean it toward your shoulder. **3.** Walk your hand back to the starting position. **4.** Repeat 8–12 times. **5.** Repeat steps 1–4 on the other side.

Perform steps 1–5, 1 time.

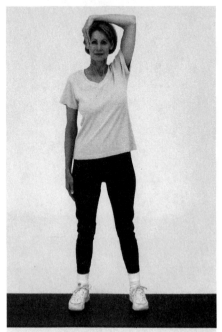

Exercise 5: Shoulder Extension

Swan Dive

PURPOSE

To stretch the muscles in the front of the shoulder, upper arm, armpit (axilla), and chest and to improve range of motion in shoulder extension.

STARTING POSITION A

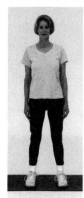

- Stand up straight
- Arms at your sides
- Feet shoulder width apart
- Knees slightly bent
- Abdominals contracted
- Lower back muscles contracted
- Shoulders down and back
- Chest lifted
- Look straight ahead

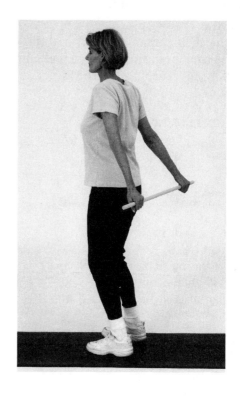

DESCRIPTION OF EXERCISE

1. Hold a dowel behind you, with your arms slightly bent, hands hip width apart (or wider if it is more comfortable for you), and palms facing your buttocks. Rest the dowel on your buttocks. **2.** Raising your arms behind you, lift the dowel off your buttocks until you feel a stretch in the front of your shoulder. As you lift, don't rock or lean forward. Keep your head still and don't shrug your shoulders or tighten your neck. **3.** Hold the stretch for 15 seconds. **4.** Slowly lower the dowel back to the starting position. **5.** Repeat 4–6 times.

Perform steps 1–5, 1 time.

Exercise 6: Pull Over

Good-Morning Stretch

PURPOSE
To stretch the armpit (axilla) and muscles in the back of the arm to improve range of motion in reaching overhead (shoulder flexion).

STARTING POSITION B

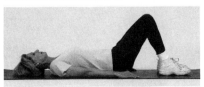

- Lie on your back
- Knees bent
- Feet flat on floor, hip width apart
- Abdominals contracted
- Small of your back pressed into the floor
- Arms straight at your sides, palms down

DESCRIPTION OF EXERCISE
1. With your arms shoulder width apart and elbows straight, grasp a dowel in front of you so that your palms face up and your thumbs point outward (not toward each other). **2.** Keeping your arms straight, inhale as you raise your arms slowly until the dowel is over your face. **3.** Exhale as you slowly lower your arms as far as you can over your head toward the floor, letting the weight of your arms stretch your armpit (axilla). Relax in this position and breathe as you hold the stretch for 15 seconds. **4.** Inhale as you raise your arms slowly until the dowel is again over your face. **5.** Repeat steps 3 and 4, 4–6 times. Don't let your back arch as you do this exercise, or the stretch will not be as effective because you will be substituting back motion for isolated arm motion.

Perform steps 1–5, 1 time.

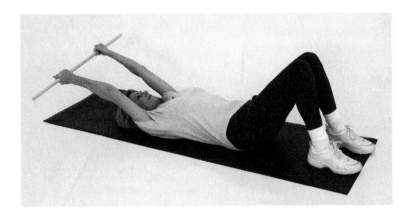

Exercise 7: Side-to-Side Arm Push

Vaudeville

PURPOSE

To stretch the armpit (axilla) and muscles along the inside of the arm and shoulder and to improve range of motion in horizontal adduction and abduction of the shoulder.

STARTING POSITION A

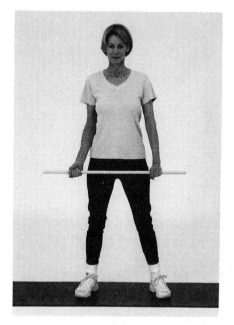

- Stand up straight
- Arms at your sides
- Feet shoulder width apart
- Knees slightly bent
- Abdominals contracted
- Lower back muscles contracted
- Shoulders down and back
- Chest lifted
- Look straight ahead

DESCRIPTION OF EXERCISE

1. With your hands slightly wider than hip width apart, hold a dowel in front of you, resting it on your thighs. The palm of your affected arm faces away from your body and the other palm faces your thigh. **2.** Without moving your trunk, move the dowel across your body toward your affected side, raising the dowel as high as possible, pushing it up toward your ear. Feel the stretch in your armpit (axilla). **3.** Hold the dowel alongside your trunk for 15 seconds. Make sure you keep your back straight and your hips facing forward (don't bend or twist your torso). **4.** Lower the dowel, then repeat the movement 4–6 times. **5.** Reverse your hand positions and repeat steps 2–4, moving the dowel toward the other side.

Perform steps 1–5, 1 time.

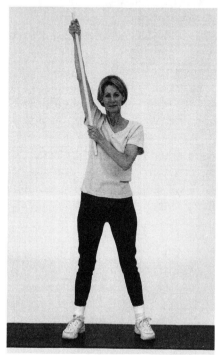

Level

I

Exercise 8: Back Scratcher

Scratching Your Back

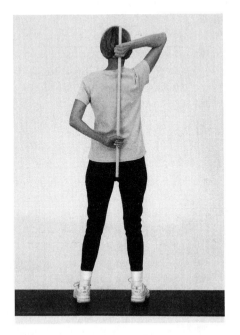

PURPOSE
To improve range of motion in external and internal rotation of the shoulder.

STARTING POSITION A

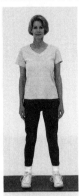

- Stand up straight
- Arms at your sides
- Feet shoulder width apart
- Knees slightly bent
- Abdominals contracted
- Lower back muscles contracted
- Shoulders down and back
- Chest lifted
- Look straight ahead

DESCRIPTION OF EXERCISE
1. Hold a dowel behind your back so that the dowel is almost vertical. Hold the dowel near the top with the hand on your unaffected side, palm facing in. Hold the dowel near the bottom with the hand on your affected side, palm facing out. **2.** Using the top hand, raise and lower the dowel to move your affected arm up and down. Make sure your movements are slow and smooth so you don't overextend the affected arm. **3.** Raise and lower the dowel 8–12 times. **4.** Reverse hand positions and repeat steps 2 and 3, 8–12 times.

Perform steps 1–4, 1 time.

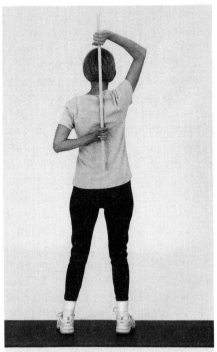

Traffic Cop

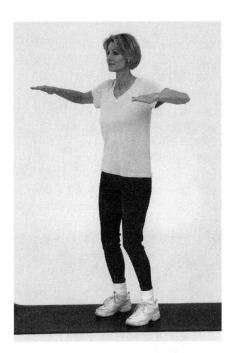

PURPOSE

To increase range of motion in external shoulder rotation, strengthen the rotator cuff, and improve stability of the shoulder joint.

STARTING POSITION A

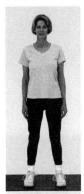

- Stand up straight
- Arms at your sides
- Feet shoulder width apart
- Knees slightly bent
- Abdominals contracted
- Lower back muscles contracted
- Shoulders down and back
- Chest lifted
- Look straight ahead

DESCRIPTION OF EXERCISE

1. Bend your elbows 90 degrees and raise your arms out to the sides at shoulder height, so that your forearms and upper arms are parallel to the floor. (Your palms will be facing the floor.) **2.** Keeping your upper arms parallel to the floor and your shoulder blades down and together, exhale as you rotate your arms upward until your forearms are perpendicular to the floor. Your upper arms remain in line with your shoulder. (Your palms will be facing forward.) **3.** Inhale as you slowly lower your arms to the starting position. Keep your back straight and your abdominals tight. Do not rock or sway. **4.** Perform 8–12 repetitions.

Perform steps 1–4, 1 time. If you are feeling tired, this exercise can be done sitting in a chair.

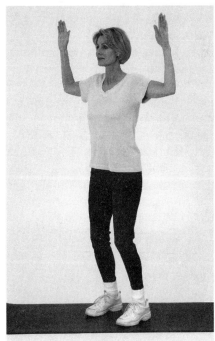

Exercise 10: Corner or Wall Chest Stretch

Spying Through a Window

PURPOSE

To stretch your chest muscles and the incision and skin across the chest wall. This will help alleviate tightness in the chest muscles, which can affect your posture by pulling the shoulder forward and giving you a hunchbacked appearance.

STARTING POSITION A

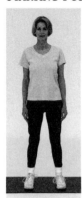

- Stand up straight
- Arms at your sides
- Feet shoulder width apart
- Knees slightly bent
- Abdominals contracted
- Lower back muscles contracted
- Shoulders down and back
- Chest lifted
- Look straight ahead

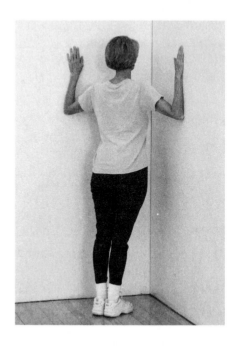

DESCRIPTION OF EXERCISE

1. Stand facing a corner, an upper arm's length away from each wall. Bend your elbows 90 degrees and raise your arms to shoulder height so that your upper arms are parallel to the floor and your palms and forearms rest on the walls. 2. Slowly lean your chest into the corner. Keep your forearms flat against the wall. 3. Hold the stretch for 15 seconds. You should feel this stretch across the front of your chest and shoulders. 4. Repeat 4–6 times.

Perform steps 1–4, 1 time.

This can also be done in a doorway.

You can vary this exercise (or find a more comfortable position) by raising or lowering your arms. This will cause you to feel the stretch across the chest wall in slightly different places. If you feel any pain, discontinue the exercise.

If a corner or doorway is not available (as in a group setting), modify the stretch by standing an upper arm's length away from the wall, with your affected side toward the wall. Raise your arm so that the upper arm is in line with your shoulder or slightly below, your elbow is bent at 90 degrees, and your forearm is perpendicular to the ground (fingertips point straight up toward the ceiling). Place your forearm on the wall with your palm flat. Keeping your forearm and palm flat against the wall, gently turn your body away from the wall. Hold for 15 seconds. Repeat 4–6 times. Repeat on the other side.

Exercise 11: Shoulder Blade Squeeze

Level

I

Chicken Wings

PURPOSE

To improve range of motion in horizontal abduction of the shoulder, improve posture by increasing muscular awareness and strength of the upper back, and reduce hunchback (kyphosis), which can occur after surgery due to tightening in the chest wall.

STARTING POSITION A

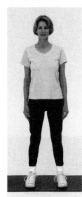

- Stand up straight
- Arms at your sides
- Feet shoulder width apart
- Knees slightly bent
- Abdominals contracted
- Lower back muscles contracted
- Shoulders down and back
- Chest lifted
- Look straight ahead

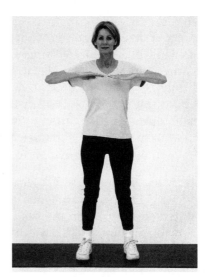

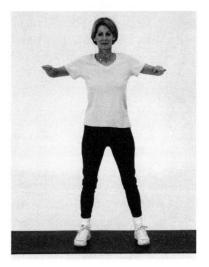

DESCRIPTION OF EXERCISE

1. Raise your arms to shoulder height or just below, bend your elbows, and touch your fingertips together in front of your chest, with your palms facing down. **2.** Pull your shoulder blades down and back (together) and hold them there as you draw your elbows back as if you could touch them together behind you. Keep your arms at the same height as your starting position as you move your elbows back. Do not shrug your shoulders up toward your ears. **3.** Hold for 5 seconds. **4.** Move your elbows forward until your fingertips are again touching in front of you. Release your shoulder blades. **5.** Repeat steps 2–4, 8–12 times. Initially per-form only 1 set of repetitions. You can build to performing 2–3 sets.

Remember to keep breathing throughout this exercise. It is imperative to avoid holding your breath during the 5-second holding time.

Level

I

Victory

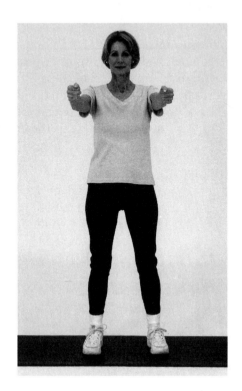

PURPOSE

To improve range of motion and begin strength work in shoulder flexion and to contract the front of the shoulder (anterior deltoid muscle) and other muscles involved in raising the arms overhead. This movement opens up the armpit (axilla), which may help clear the shoulder lymph pathway and thus help the lymph to flow.

STARTING POSITION A

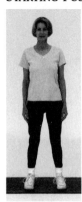

- Stand up straight
- Arms at your sides
- Feet shoulder width apart
- Knees slightly bent
- Abdominals contracted
- Lower back muscles contracted
- Shoulders down and back
- Chest lifted
- Look straight ahead

DESCRIPTION OF EXERCISE

1. With palms facing in, bend your elbows slightly and exhale as you raise both arms in front of you. Go only as high as the affected shoulder will let you. If you are performing the exercise without weights, you can progress to raising your arms as high as they can go to increase your range of motion. (Note that if you perform this exercise with weights—as you will in higher levels—you will raise your arms only to shoulder height.) **2.** Inhale as you lower both arms slowly. **3.** Repeat 8–12 times. Initially perform only 1 set of repetitions. You can build to performing 2–3 sets.

If you have pain or pinching in the shoulder with this exercise, raise your arm only in your pain-free range. If any motion is painful, do not do the exercise.

Exercise 13: Arm Raise to the Side

Level

I

Eagle Flapping Its Wings

PURPOSE

To increase range of motion and begin strength work in shoulder abduction and to contract the middle portion of the shoulder muscle (medial deltoid) to help lymph move through alternative pathways.

STARTING POSITION A

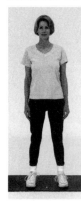

- Stand up straight
- Arms at your sides
- Feet shoulder width apart
- Knees slightly bent
- Abdominals contracted
- Lower back muscles contracted
- Shoulders down and back
- Chest lifted
- Look straight ahead

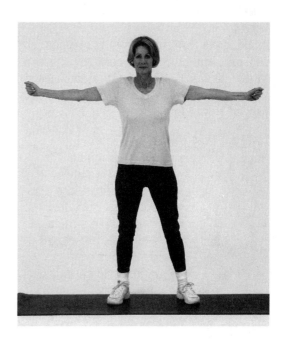

DESCRIPTION OF EXERCISE

1. With your palms facing forward and your arms slightly bent, exhale as you raise both arms out to the sides until they are parallel to the floor. Keep your shoulder blades down and together; do not shrug your shoulders. **2.** Inhale as you slowly lower both arms. **3.** Repeat 8–12 times. Initially perform only 1 set of repetitions. You can build to performing 2–3 sets.

Level

I

| Exercise 14: Biceps Curl |

Popeye

PURPOSE

To work the front muscle of the upper arm (biceps) and help with bending the arm (elbow flexion). Working the muscles of the hand and elbow can help move lymph trapped in the forearm.

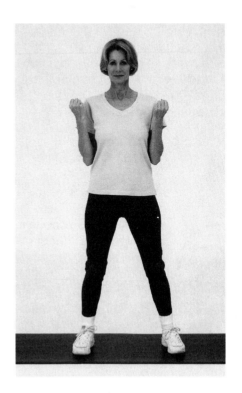

STARTING POSITION A

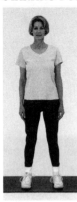

- Stand up straight
- Arms at your sides
- Feet shoulder width apart
- Knees slightly bent
- Abdominals contracted
- Lower back muscles contracted
- Shoulders down and back
- Chest lifted
- Look straight ahead

DESCRIPTION OF EXERCISE

1. Turn your palms so they face forward, then close both hands in a loose fist. Keep your elbows close to your sides and under your shoulders, your shoulder blades down and back, and your back straight. **2.** Contracting your front upper arm muscles (biceps) throughout the motion, exhale and slowly raise your fists toward your shoulders. Imagine your elbows as pivot points that allow you to move your forearms up and down. **3.** Inhale and slowly lower your fists to the starting position. **4.** Repeat 8–12 times. Initially perform only 1 set of repetitions. You can build to performing 2–3 sets.

Exercise 15: Arm Extension (Triceps)

Quarterback Throwing a Football

PURPOSE

To work the back muscle of the upper arm (triceps) and help with straightening the arm (elbow extension). Working the muscles of the hand and elbow can help move lymph trapped in the forearm.

STARTING POSITION B

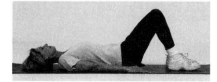

- Lie on your back
- Knees bent
- Feet flat on floor, hip width apart
- Abdominals contracted
- Small of your back pressed into the floor
- Arms straight at your sides, palms down

DESCRIPTION OF EXERCISE

1. Raise your right arm straight up toward the ceiling, with your palm facing in. **2.** Place your left hand below your right elbow to support the working arm. **3.** Inhale as you bend your right elbow and lower your forearm toward your body. Your elbow should point straight up toward the ceiling, and your right palm should end up at ear level. **4.** Contract your triceps and exhale as you slowly straighten your elbow until your arm has returned to the starting position (straight up toward the ceiling). **5.** Repeat the bending and straightening motion 8–12 times. **6.** Repeat on the other side. Initially perform only 1 set of repetitions. You can build to performing 2–3 sets.

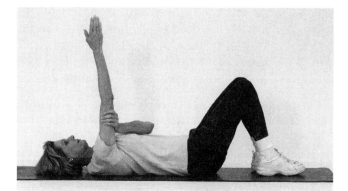

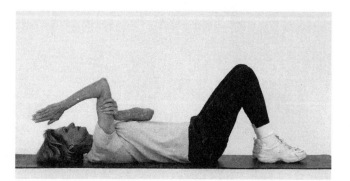

Level
I

Exercise 16: Serratus Reach

Reaching for the Stars

PURPOSE
To strengthen the serratus anterior muscle of the shoulder girdle, which holds the shoulder blade against the back, and to prevent feelings of weakness in the arm when reaching in front of you.

STARTING POSITION B

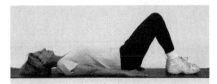

- Lie on your back
- Knees bent
- Feet flat on floor, hip width apart
- Abdominals contracted
- Small of your back pressed into the floor
- Arms straight at your sides, palms down

DESCRIPTION OF EXERCISE
1. Raise both arms so that they are pointing up toward the ceiling (perpendicular to the floor), with your palms facing your feet. **2.** Exhale as you reach for the ceiling by raising your arms as high as you can, lifting your shoulders off the floor. Keep your elbows straight. **3.** Hold your arms up for 5 seconds. **4.** Inhale as you lower your arms back to the starting position. **5.** Repeat the reaching and lowering motion 8–12 times. Initially perform only 1 set of repetitions. You can build to performing 2–3 sets.

Note that your head and back stay on the floor; only your shoulders lift up as you reach toward the ceiling.

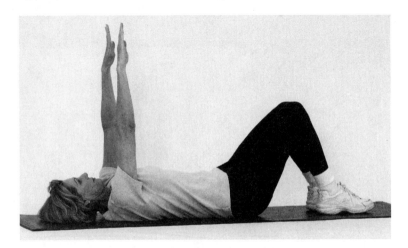

Exercise 17: Lower Back (Floor Work)

Bridging

PURPOSE

To strengthen the lower back and develop core body strength. This exercise is particularly beneficial for those who have had a TRAM flap. Additionally, it can help improve posture, which can be adversely affected by mastectomy and reconstructive surgery. With any of the back exercises, stop if you feel any pain.

MAIN MUSCLES WORKED

Lower back (erector spinae), back of thighs (hamstrings), and buttocks (gluteals).

STARTING POSITION B

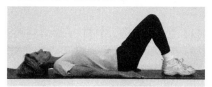

- Lie on your back
- Knees bent
- Feet flat on floor, hip width apart
- Abdominals contracted
- Small of your back pressed into the floor
- Arms straight at your sides, palms down

DESCRIPTION OF EXERCISE

1. Raise your hips (pelvis) off the floor by contracting your abdominals, lower back, and buttocks until your body forms a straight line from your kneecaps and thighs to your chin. Be sure to keep your shoulders and upper back in contact with the floor. **2.** Keeping your pelvis level, hold the straight-line position for 5 seconds. **3.** Lower your hips back to the floor. **4.** Repeat 8–12 times. Initially perform only 1 set of repetitions. You can build to performing 2–3 sets.

Remember to breathe consistently throughout the exercise. Do not hold your breath.

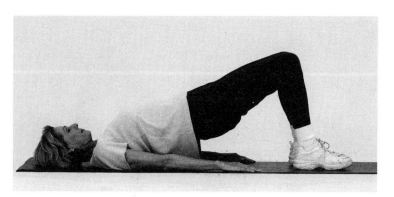

Level

I

Strong to the Core

PURPOSE

To strengthen the abdominals and provide core body strength. This exercise can help relieve lower back pain and improve posture (which can be adversely affected by mastectomy and reconstructive surgery) by strengthening the abdominals and reducing swayback.

MAIN MUSCLES WORKED

Abdominals and buttocks (gluteals).

STARTING POSITION B

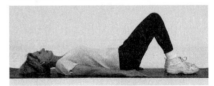

- Lie on your back
- Knees bent
- Feet flat on floor, hip width apart
- Abdominals contracted
- Small of your back pressed into the floor
- Arms straight at your sides, palms down

DESCRIPTION OF EXERCISE

1. Flatten your lower back into the floor by contracting your abdominals and buttocks at the same time. If you have trouble with the motion, think of pressing the small of your back into the floor as if you were trying to squish a grape. **2.** Hold the position for 5 seconds and then return to the starting position. **3.** Repeat 8–12 times. Initially perform only 1 set of repetitions. You can build to performing 2–3 sets.

This exercise can also be done with your legs straight or while standing (place your back against a wall if you need support while doing this exercise in a standing position).

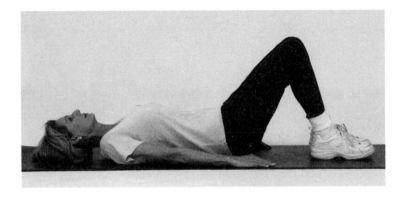

Exercise 19: Abdominal Stretch   Level I

Lion

PURPOSE
To stretch the abdominals and lower back. This exercise is especially helpful for those who have had a TRAM flap and are having trouble with their posture and lower back pain.

MAIN MUSCLES WORKED
Abdominals and lower back (erector spinae).

STARTING POSITION
See "Description of Exercise."

DESCRIPTION OF EXERCISE
1. Lie facedown on the floor. Bend your arms and place your forearms flat on the floor, with your palms near your head. Hold your elbows close by your side. If you need to, put a pillow under your chest and stomach for cushioning and support. **2.** Exhale as you raise yourself up onto your forearms. Keep your forearms flat on the floor, supporting your upper body. Keep your elbows against your body and directly in line with your shoulders. Try to let your back sag and stay relaxed. **3.** Pause for 5 seconds, making sure to breathe. **4.** Slowly lower yourself back to the floor. **5.** Repeat 8–12 times.

Perform steps 1–5, 1 time.

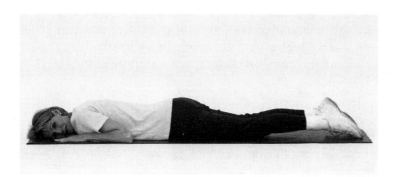

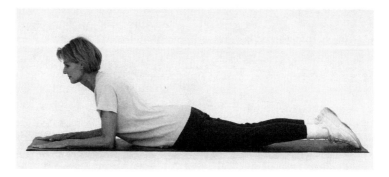

Level

I

Swami

PURPOSE

To stretch the armpit (axilla) and back of the arm and to improve range of motion in shoulder flexion. If you have any pain in your affected arm, do not do this exercise.

STARTING POSITION C

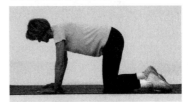

- On hands and knees
- Hands directly beneath shoulders (fingers face forward)
- Arms straight but not locked
- Knees shoulder width apart
- Head and neck a natural extension of the spine

DESCRIPTION OF EXERCISE

1. Make sure most of your weight is on your legs and your unaffected arm. **2.** Slowly move your hips back and rest your buttocks on your heels as you lower your head toward the floor (between your arms). You should feel a gentle stretch in your shoulders. **3.** Hold this position for 5 seconds. **4.** Return to the starting position. **5.** Repeat 8–12 times.

Perform steps 1–5, 1 time.

For an extra challenge, first inhale, then, as you exhale, gradually walk your fingers farther out in front of you while keeping your buttocks on your heels.

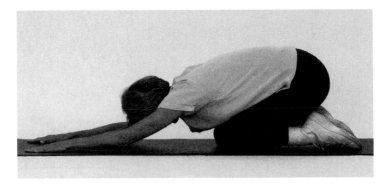

Exercise 21: End-to-End Stretch

Elongation

PURPOSE
To stretch and relax the body from head to toe.

MAIN MUSCLES WORKED
Whole body.

STARTING POSITION D

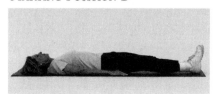

- Lie on your back
- Legs straight
- Arms straight at your sides, palms down

DESCRIPTION OF EXERCISE
1. Reach your arms out on the floor over your head as straight as you comfortably can. **2.** Inhale deeply and think relaxing thoughts. **3.** Exhale and reach for the wall behind you with your arms and for the wall in front of you with your feet, as if someone were pulling you from end to end. **4.** At the end of your exhalation, relax your entire body. You will be lying flat on the floor with your arms overhead. Breathe in and out several times. **5.** Repeat 8–12 times.

Perform steps 1–5, 1 time.

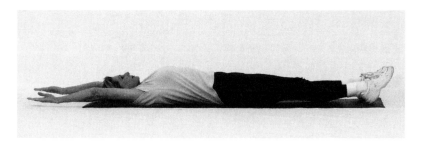

Remember, advance to Level II only when you satisfy these conditions:

- You can perform either the number of sets and repetitions listed for each exercise, or two to three sets of 8–12 repetitions for all exercises in Level I.
- You have achieved range of motion on your affected side that is similar to your unaffected side.
- You have not experienced any negative responses in your affected arm (including swelling, achiness, numbness, redness, tissue texture change).
- You feel ready.

Continue to perform your Level I range-of-motion exercises even after you progress to the higher levels.

Level II

Level II begins the conditioning of the upper and lower body. These exercises are functional in nature and are designed to strengthen all the major muscle groups, although emphasis is placed on the upper body. The exercises incorporate balance and postural training, as you must maintain proper posture and positioning throughout them. Specific abdominal and lower back exercises are also included.

Begin with one set of 8–12 repetitions and progress to two to three sets of 8–12 repetitions. Some of these exercises include the use of a dowel, 1- to 5-pound weights, or an exercise band. Follow the precautions in Chapter 3 (page 35), and review "Points to Remember When Performing All Exercises" on page 46.

You may advance to Level III when you can do two to three sets of 8–12 repetitions of all the exercises. Do not advance if you do not feel up to it. If you experience pain or loss of range of motion, stop exercising and see your doctor.

Remember, your arm's response to exercise is your ultimate indicator for progressing in the program. If you feel pain or notice redness, change in skin texture, or swelling, stop exercising and call your doctor immediately. If you are given the OK to continue, reduce the number of repetitions and the resistance you are using.

Level II Exercises

	TECHNICAL NAME	ANALOGY NAME
Exercise 1	"Lat" Pull Down with Band	Pose of Strength
Exercise 2	Quarter Squat with Leg Lifts	Marionette
Exercise 3	Wall Push-ups	Pushing All My Worries Away
Exercise 4	Plié	Curtsy
Exercise 5	Chest Squeeze	Praying
Exercise 6	Exercise Ball Squat with Frontal Arm Raise	Riding a Motorcycle
Exercise 7	Shoulder Blade Squeeze with Optional Band	Chicken Wings
Exercise 8	Hamstring Curls with Optional Weights	Balancing Act
Exercise 9	Lying Pull Over with Optional Weight	Playing with a Baby
Exercise 10	Standing Knee Raise	Stork
Exercise 11	Shoulder Shrugs	I Don't Know!

Exercise 12	Standing Calf Raise	Looking over the Fence
Exercise 13	Internal Rotation (Shoulder/Rotator Cuff)	Pulling the Door Shut
Exercise 14	External Rotation (Shoulder/Rotator Cuff)	Opening the Door
Exercise 15	Side Arm Raise with Shoulder Rotation	Emptying the Can
Exercise 16	Biceps Curl with Weights	Popeye
Exercise 17	One-Arm Extension with Weight	Casting a Fishing Line
Exercise 18	Hand Rotations with Dowel	Rolling Dough
Exercise 19	Lower Back (Floor Work)	Modified Superwoman
Exercise 20	Lower Back (Floor Work)	Superwoman
Exercise 21	Lower Back (Floor Work)	Bridging
Exercise 22	Abdominals (Floor Work)	Bending in Half
Exercise 23	Abdominals (Standing)	Cheerleader

Exercise 1: "Lat" Pull Down with Band

Pose of Strength

PURPOSE
To strengthen the back muscles while stretching the incision and skin across the chest wall. This will help alleviate tight chest muscles and strengthen weak back muscles, which can impair your posture by pulling the shoulder forward and rounding the back, giving a hunchbacked appearance.

MAIN MUSCLES WORKED
Back (latissimus dorsi, rhomboids, teres major, middle and lower trapezius), back of shoulders (posterior deltoid), and front of upper arms (biceps).

STARTING POSITION A

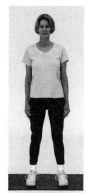

- Stand up straight
- Arms at your sides
- Feet shoulder width apart
- Knees slightly bent
- Abdominals contracted
- Lower back muscles contracted
- Shoulders down and back
- Chest lifted
- Look straight ahead

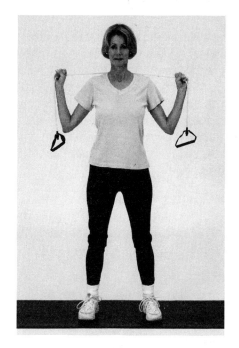

DESCRIPTION OF EXERCISE
1. Hold an exercise band stretched taut between your hands and raise your arms above your head, keeping your elbows slightly bent. Your palms should face forward, and your hands should be shoulder width apart. The tension in the exercise band should be low, not painful. 2. Pull your shoulder blades down and together, bend your elbows, and lower your arms until your hands come down just below your shoulders. The band will come down behind your head. Your arms and hands should remain in line with the sides of your body; your elbows should point out to your sides, then down toward the floor as you lower your arms. (Think of a chicken squeezing its wings together.) Keep your shoulder blades pulled down and together throughout the movement. Do not shrug your shoulders. Keep your head up and your back straight. Do not rock or sway. 3. Hold for 5 seconds. 4. Return to the starting position. 5. Perform 8–12 repetitions.

Remember to keep breathing throughout this exercise.

If you perform this exercise on a weight machine, do not pull the bar down behind your head. Keep your head still and aligned with your spine.

Level II

Exercise 2: Quarter Squat with Leg Lifts

Marionette

PURPOSE
To improve posture and balance, strengthen and stabilize the torso, and improve lower body range of motion. You will use your abdominals and buttocks to stabilize your torso, which will help protect your lower back from injury. You will also use the muscles involved in pelvic stabilization and everyday activities such as sitting, standing, and walking.

MAIN MUSCLES WORKED
Buttocks (gluteals), back of thighs (hamstrings), front of thighs (quadriceps), and hips (abductors).

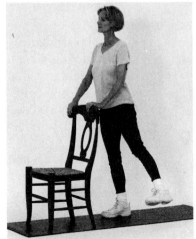

STARTING POSITION A

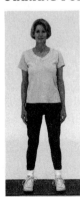

- Stand up straight
- Arms at your sides
- Feet shoulder width apart
- Knees slightly bent
- Abdominals contracted
- Lower back muscles contracted
- Shoulders down and back
- Chest lifted
- Look straight ahead

DESCRIPTION OF EXERCISE
1. Place your hands on the back of a chair for support. Bend your knees so that you squat down into a quarter squat. Be sure to keep your knees over your feet and not to let them go past your toes. This will help protect your knees from injury. Keep your shoulders and hips square, your torso upright, your spine straight, and your head up. **2.** Exhale as you straighten your legs and shift your weight onto your right foot.

Tighten your buttocks and lift your left leg out to the side, no higher than 45 degrees. Keep a slight bend in the right (supporting) leg, but don't bend your torso to the side as you lift. **3.** Inhale as you return to the starting squat position. **4.** Repeat on the other side. **5.** Perform 6 repetitions on each side, for a total of 12 repetitions. Gradually increase the number of sets as you feel more comfortable with the exercise.

Exercise 3: Wall Push-ups

Pushing All My Worries Away

PURPOSE
To strengthen the muscles of the chest wall and improve upper body range of motion to help you perform everyday activities and develop muscle symmetry.

MAIN MUSCLES WORKED
Chest (pectorals), front of shoulders (anterior deltoids), back of upper arms (triceps), and a shoulder girdle muscle (serratus anterior).

STARTING POSITION A

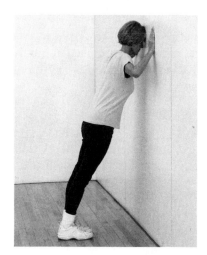

• Stand up straight
• Arms at your sides
• Feet shoulder width apart
• Knees slightly bent
• Abdominals contracted
• Lower back muscles contracted
• Shoulders down and back
• Chest lifted
• Look straight ahead

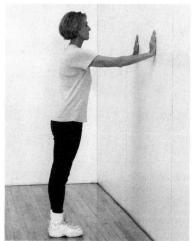

DESCRIPTION OF EXERCISE
1. Stand facing a wall with your feet shoulder width apart and about 15–18 inches from the wall. (The farther back you stand, the harder you'll have to work.) Place your palms flat on the wall about shoulder width apart and slightly above your shoulders. Bend your arms and place your forehead on the wall between your hands. (Your hands should be level with your head.) **2.** Exhale and push yourself away from the wall by straightening your elbows. Push out until your arms are straight without locking your elbows. Try to contract your chest muscles while you press away from the wall. (This is a diffi- cult contraction for many people.) **3.** Inhale as you return to the starting position by lowering yourself toward the wall and bending your elbows. Throughout the exercise, keep your palms in contact with the wall, feet flat, knees slightly bent, and back straight. Be sure to contract your abdominals and squeeze your buttocks to stabilize your torso. Push with your arms and chest; don't lift with your back. **4.** Repeat 8–12 times.

Exercise 4: Plié

Curtsy

PURPOSE
To improve balance, improve torso stability, and strengthen muscles involved in everyday activities such as sitting, standing, and walking.

MAIN MUSCLES WORKED
Front of thighs (quadriceps), back of thighs (hamstrings), buttocks (gluteals), and some inner thighs (adductors).

STARTING POSITION E

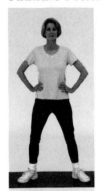

- Stand up straight
- Hands on hips
- Feet wider than shoulder width apart
- Toes turned out slightly to the side
- Knees slightly bent
- Abdominals contracted
- Lower back muscles contracted
- Shoulders down and back
- Chest lifted
- Look straight ahead

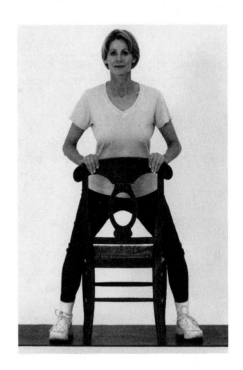

DESCRIPTION OF EXERCISE
1. Assume the starting position, with your legs straddling the seat of a chair and your hands resting on the back of the chair for support. Keep your abdominals and gluteals contracted throughout the exercise. 2. Inhale as you bend your knees and lower your torso straight down until you are almost sitting on the chair. Keep your abdominals contracted, your rib cage lifted, and your torso over your hips. Do not arch your back or bend forward or backward. Make sure your knees do not go past your toes. 3. Exhale as you straighten your legs and return to the starting position. 4. Perform 8–12 repetitions.

Exercise 5: Chest Squeeze

Praying

PURPOSE

To strengthen the chest wall, improve muscle symmetry, promote muscle awareness, and improve the ability to perform daily activities involving the upper body.

MAIN MUSCLES WORKED

Chest (pectorals) and shoulders (deltoids).

STARTING POSITION A

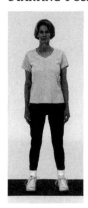

- Stand up straight
- Arms at your sides
- Feet shoulder width apart
- Knees slightly bent
- Abdominals contracted
- Lower back muscles contracted
- Shoulders down and back
- Chest lifted
- Look straight ahead

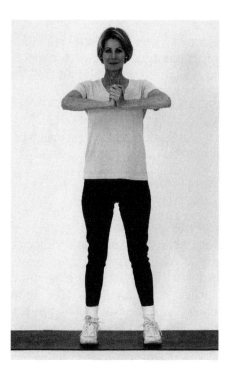

DESCRIPTION OF EXERCISE

1. Clasp your hands in front of you, raise your arms to shoulder height or just below, and bend your elbows at a 90-degree angle. **2.** Pulling your shoulder blades down and together and holding them there, push your hands together (against each other) so that you feel the muscle contraction in your chest. **3.** Hold for 5 seconds, breathing normally, and then relax, keeping your hands and arms in the step 1 position. **4.** Repeat 8–12 times.

Remember to keep breathing throughout this exercise. It is imperative to avoid holding your breath during an isometric exercise.

Level

II

| **Exercise 6: Exercise Ball Squat with Frontal Arm Raise** |

Riding a Motorcycle

PURPOSE
To improve lower body strength, increase range of motion in the shoulder, and improve shoulder strength and stability.

MAIN MUSCLES WORKED
Buttocks (gluteals), front of thighs (quadriceps), back of thighs (hamstrings), and front of shoulders (anterior deltoids).

STARTING POSITION
See "Description of Exercise."

DESCRIPTION OF EXERCISE
1. Stand near the wall with a rubber exercise ball in the small of your back and against the wall. Walk your legs out about 18 inches, keeping your feet shoulder width apart and your toes pointing forward. Your arms should hang by your sides, with your palms facing your thighs. **2.** Inhale as you press back firmly against the ball and lower your torso by bending your knees. Go as low as you comfortably can, but no lower than with your knees bent at a 90-degree angle. Keep your knees over your feet—not beyond your toes. (Try to keep them over your ankles.) As you lower yourself, raise your arms out in front of you to shoulder height. **3.** Exhale as you straighten your legs and lower your arms back to your sides. Do not lock your knees or elbows. Keep your head and neck straight and look forward. **4.** Repeat 8–12 times.

If it feels more natural to you, breathe in the opposite pattern from that described above.

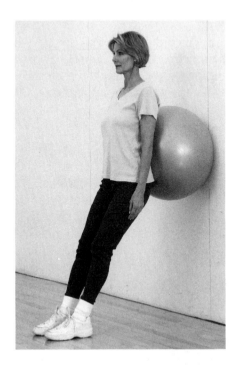

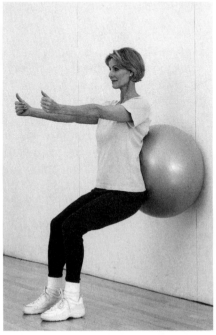

Exercise 7: Shoulder Blade Squeeze with Optional Band

Level

II

Chicken Wings

PURPOSE
To improve range of motion in horizontal abduction of the shoulder, improve posture by increasing muscular awareness and strength of the upper back, and reduce hunchback (kyphosis), which can occur after surgery due to tightening in the chest wall.

MAIN MUSCLES WORKED
Upper back (rhomboids), mid-back (middle and lower trapezius), back of shoulders (posterior deltoids), and rotator cuffs (teres minor, infraspinatus).

STARTING POSITION A

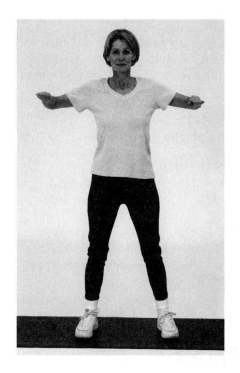

- Stand up straight
- Arms at your sides
- Feet shoulder width apart
- Knees slightly bent
- Abdominals contracted
- Lower back muscles contracted
- Shoulders down and back
- Chest lifted
- Look straight ahead

DESCRIPTION OF EXERCISE
1. Raise your arms to shoulder height or just below, bend your elbows, and touch your fingertips together in front of your chest, with your palms facing down (see top photo on page 77). **2.** Pull your shoulder blades down and back (together) and hold them there as you draw your elbows back as if you could touch them together behind you. Keep your arms at the same height as your starting position as you move your elbows back. Do not shrug your shoulders up toward your ears. **3.** Hold for 5 seconds. **4.** Move your elbows forward until your fingertips are again touching in front of you. Release your shoulder blades. **5.** Repeat steps 2–4, 8–12 times.

To add resistance, hold an exercise band with your hands about shoulder width apart. If you are unable to draw your elbows back with good form, the tension is too great. Place your hands farther apart on the band to decrease the tension. The tension should be low and not cause any pain.

Remember to keep breathing throughout this exercise. It is imperative to avoid holding your breath during the 5-second hold time.

Exercise 8: Hamstring Curls with Optional Weights

Balancing Act

PURPOSE
To improve posture and balance and to increase leg strength, which is vital to performing everyday activities and maintaining functional independence.

MAIN MUSCLES WORKED
Back of thighs (hamstrings).

STARTING POSITION F

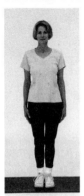

- Stand up straight
- Arms at your sides
- Feet together
- Knees slightly bent
- Abdominals contracted
- Lower back muscles contracted
- Shoulders down and back
- Chest lifted
- Look straight ahead

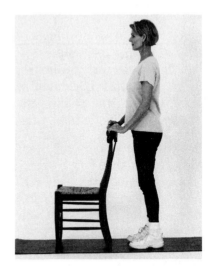

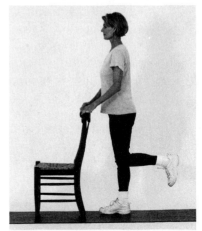

DESCRIPTION OF EXERCISE
1. Hold on to the back of a chair for balance. **2.** Keeping your thighs parallel, exhale and bend one knee, lifting the heel toward the buttocks. The heel does not need to come any closer than 45 degrees from the buttocks. Keep your foot flexed throughout the motion (don't point your toes). Keep the knee of the bent leg centered underneath the hip, next to the stationary knee. (If the thigh moves backward, you may place undue stress on the knee.) Focus on the muscle contraction in the back of the upper leg as you bend the knee. Only the knee joint is moving. Throughout the exercise, contract your abdominals and buttocks, keep your pelvis level and still, lift your rib cage, look straight ahead, keep the knee of the support leg slightly bent, keep your foot flexed, and keep your torso straight and upright (do not bend at the hips or waist). **3.** Pause for a second. **4.** Inhale and slowly straighten your knee and return to the starting position. **5.** Repeat 8–12 times. **6.** Repeat the exercise with the other leg.

For added resistance, you can wear 1- to 5-pound ankle weights while performing this exercise.

Exercise 9: Lying Pull Over with Optional Weight

Level

II

Playing with a Baby

PURPOSE

To improve torso stability, increase muscle symmetry, and increase upper body range of motion and strength, especially following axillary node dissection.

MAIN MUSCLES WORKED

Back (latissimus dorsi), upper back (rhomboids), chest (upper pectorals), a shoulder girdle muscle (serratus anterior), and back of upper arms (triceps).

STARTING POSITION B

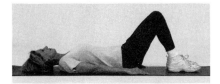

- Lie on your back
- Knees bent
- Feet flat on floor, hip width apart
- Abdominals contracted
- Small of your back pressed into the floor
- Arms straight at your sides, palms down

DESCRIPTION OF EXERCISE

1. Extend your arms toward the ceiling above your chest and clasp your hands together in the air. **2.** Inhale deeply as you move your arms over your head toward the floor until you feel a mild stretch in your chest. Keep your arms straight (with a slight bend in your elbows), your buttocks and lower back pressed down into the floor, your abdominals contracted, and your upper arms close to your head. **3.** Exhale as you pull your shoulder blades down and back (together) and contract your chest muscles and raise your arms back to the starting position. Focus on your back and chest muscles to perform the movement. **4.** Repeat 8–12 times.

If you have been cleared by your doctor and feel ready, you can hold a 1- to 5-pound weight between your hands.

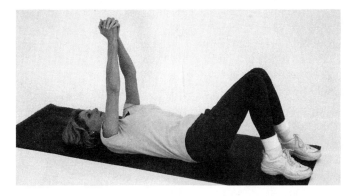

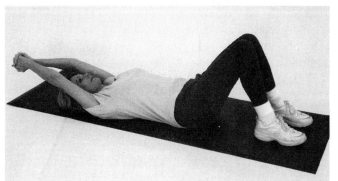

Level

II

Exercise 10: Standing Knee Raise

Stork

PURPOSE
To increase torso stability, improve posture, and increase hip flexor strength.

MAIN MUSCLES WORKED
Hip flexors.

STARTING POSITION A

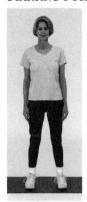

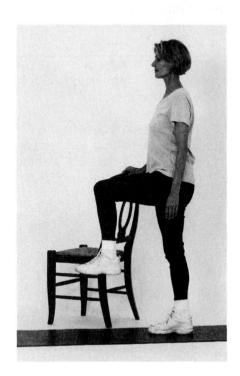

- Stand up straight
- Arms at your sides
- Feet shoulder width apart
- Knees slightly bent
- Abdominals contracted
- Lower back muscles contracted
- Shoulders down and back
- Chest lifted
- Look straight ahead

DESCRIPTION OF EXERCISE
1. Stand next to a chair for balance. **2.** Exhale and bend one knee at a 90-degree angle in front of you as if lifting the upper thigh toward your abdomen. The knee of the moving leg does not need to come higher than hip level. Keep your pelvis level and still. As the exercise becomes easier, hold this position for 3–5 seconds. **3.** Inhale and slowly straighten and lower your leg to the starting position. Rest for only a second before repeating the movement so that the muscles do not relax completely. **4.** Perform 8–12 repetitions. **5.** Repeat with the other leg.

For added resistance, you can wear 1- to 5-pound ankle weights while performing this exercise.

Exercise 11: Shoulder Shrugs

Level

II

I Don't Know!

PURPOSE
To increase upper back strength.

MAIN MUSCLES WORKED
Upper back (trapezius).

STARTING POSITION A

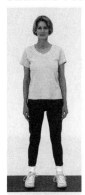

- Stand up straight
- Arms at your sides
- Feet shoulder width apart
- Knees slightly bent
- Abdominals contracted
- Lower back muscles
  contracted
- Shoulders down and back
- Chest lifted
- Look straight ahead

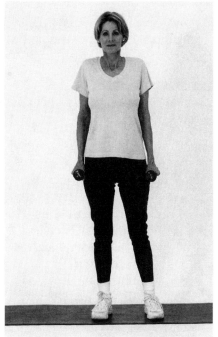

DESCRIPTION OF EXERCISE
1. Hold a 1- to 5-pound weight in each hand and let your arms hang at your sides with your palms facing your body. Do not lock your elbows. Do not rock or sway as you perform the movement. **2.** Exhale as you shrug your shoulders up toward your ears. **3.** Hold for 3–5 seconds. **4.** Inhale as you slowly lower your shoulders. Control the lowering motion. **5.** Repeat 8–12 times.

Level
II

| **Exercise 12: Standing Calf Raise** |

Looking over the Fence

PURPOSE
To improve balance by strengthening the muscles of the lower leg and improving ankle stability.

MAIN MUSCLES WORKED
Back of calf (mainly gastrocnemius and some soleus).

STARTING POSITION A

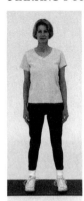

- Stand up straight
- Arms at your sides
- Feet shoulder width apart
- Knees slightly bent
- Abdominals contracted
- Lower back muscles contracted
- Shoulders down and back
- Chest lifted
- Look straight ahead

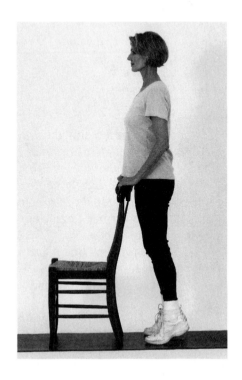

DESCRIPTION OF EXERCISE
1. Hold on to a chair or put one hand against a wall for balance. **2.** Exhale and raise up on your toes as high as you can without your ankles rolling inward or outward. Feel the contraction in your calf muscles. **3.** Inhale and lower yourself by putting your heels back down on the floor. Make sure you don't bounce up and down. Use controlled, rhythmical movements to isolate your calf muscles. **4.** Repeat 8–12 times.

As the exercise becomes easier, hold the contraction in step 2 for 3–5 seconds and don't place the heel all the way down to the ground in step 3.

When you feel stronger, perform the exercise one foot at a time. Raise one foot off the floor and rest it against your other ankle, or simply bend your leg to hold it out of the way as you raise and lower yourself on your other foot. Repeat 8–12 times with each leg.

If you have access to stairs, you can challenge yourself further and get a greater stretch in your calves and achilles tendons by standing on the balls of your feet at the edge of a step and performing the same exercise. Press your heel down until you feel a good stretch.

Exercise 13: Internal Rotation (Shoulder/Rotator Cuff)

Pulling the Door Shut

PURPOSE

To increase range of motion in shoulder rotation, strengthen the rotator cuff, and improve stability of the shoulder joint.

MAIN MUSCLES WORKED

Chest (pectoralis major), back (latissimus dorsi and teres major), rotator cuff (subscapularis), and front of shoulder (anterior deltoid).

STARTING POSITION

See "Description of Exercise."

DESCRIPTION OF EXERCISE

1. Lie on your right side on the floor and bend your knees so that they are in front of you to provide support. Keep your left knee on top of your right. Place a pillow (or equivalent) under your head for support so that your head stays aligned with your spine. Rest your left arm on your side. 2. Stretch your right arm straight out on the floor in front of you, palm toward the ceiling, and bend the elbow at a 90-degree angle to bring your upper arm back next to your side, with your elbow near your waist. (Keep your arm on the floor.) If you have been cleared by your doctor and feel ready, hold a 1- to 5-pound weight in your right hand. 3. Exhale and rotate your forearm toward the ceiling, leading with the palm. Keep your upper arm on the floor. Keep your wrist straight. 4. Inhale and return to the starting position. 5. Repeat 8–12 times. 6. Repeat on the other side.

If you choose to use a weight, as shown in the photograph, begin with 1 to 2 pounds.

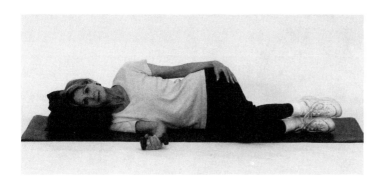

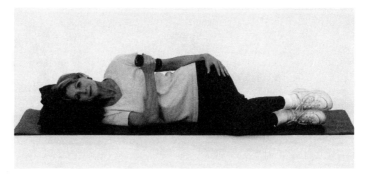

Exercise 14: External Rotation (Shoulder/Rotator Cuff)

Opening the Door

PURPOSE
To increase range of motion in shoulder rotation, strengthen the rotator cuff, and improve stability of the shoulder joint.

MAIN MUSCLES WORKED
Rotator cuff (infraspinatus and teres minor) and back of the shoulder (posterior deltoid).

STARTING POSITION
See "Description of Exercise."

DESCRIPTION OF EXERCISE
1. Lie on your right side on the floor and bend your knees so that they are in front of you to provide support. Keep your left knee on top of your right. Support your head with your right arm. **2.** Bend the elbow of your left arm at a 90-degree angle and rest your elbow on your hip. Your forearm should be parallel to the floor. Your hand should be in a loose fist, palm toward the floor. **3.** Exhale and rotate your forearm toward the ceiling, leading with the back of your hand. Your elbow stays on your hip, and your upper arm stays by your side. Keep your wrist straight. **4.** Inhale and return to the starting position. **5.** Repeat 8–12 times. **6.** Repeat on the other side.

If you choose to use a weight, as shown in the photograph, begin with 1 to 2 pounds.

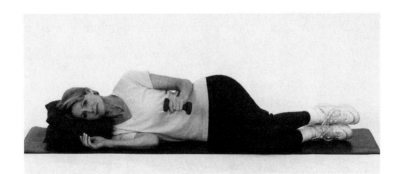

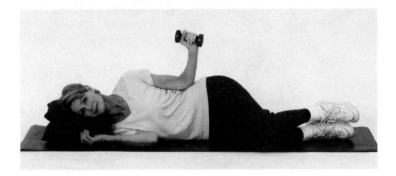

Exercise 15: Side Arm Raise with Shoulder Rotation

Emptying the Can

PURPOSE
To increase range of motion in shoulder rotation, strengthen the rotator cuff and shoulders, and improve stability of the shoulder joint.

MAIN MUSCLES WORKED
Shoulder (deltoid) and a rotator cuff muscle (supraspinatus).

STARTING POSITION A

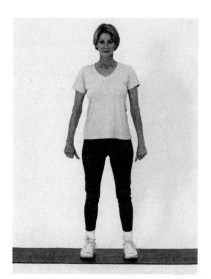

- Stand up straight
- Arms at your sides
- Feet shoulder width apart
- Knees slightly bent
- Abdominals contracted
- Lower back muscles contracted
- Shoulders down and back
- Chest lifted
- Look straight ahead

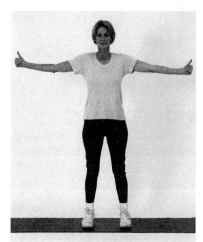

DESCRIPTION OF EXERCISE
1. Start with your arms hanging at your sides and your hands resting on the sides of your legs. 2. Exhale as you slowly and carefully raise your arms up and out to your sides. As you lift, keep your elbows slightly bent and your thumbs pointing down as if you were emptying a can. Keep your shoulder blades anchored down and back. Do not rock or swing as you perform the movement. 3. When your arms are at shoulder height, rotate them so that your thumbs point up (possibly slightly to the back). Your upper arms stay parallel to the ground; the movement comes only from rotation in the shoulder joints. 4. Return to the starting position, with your palms rest-ing on the sides of your legs. 5. Perform 8–12 repetitions.

Start with no weights and progress slowly. To add resistance, hold 1- to 5-pound weights in your hands. If you feel any pain or discomfort with weights, do not use them.

Level
II

Exercise 16: Biceps Curl with Weights

Popeye

PURPOSE
To increase upper arm strength for performing everyday activities involving pulling motions. The exercise also will help strengthen muscles used for carrying.

MAIN MUSCLES WORKED
Front of upper arms (biceps).

STARTING POSITION A

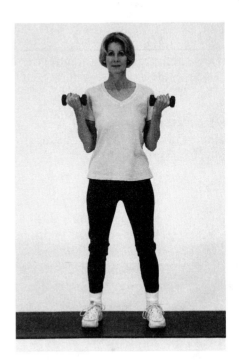

- Stand up straight
- Arms at your sides
- Feet shoulder width apart
- Knees slightly bent
- Abdominals contracted
- Lower back muscles contracted
- Shoulders down and back
- Chest lifted
- Look straight ahead

DESCRIPTION OF EXERCISE
1. Hold a 1- to 5-pound weight in each hand and hang your arms straight down at your sides, with your palms facing forward. Keep your elbows close to your sides and under your shoulders, your shoulder blades down and back, and your back straight. If you have lower back problems, stand with your back against a wall for support. 2. Contracting your front upper arm muscles (biceps) throughout the motion, exhale and slowly raise the weights toward your shoulders by bending your elbows. Imagine your elbows as pivot points that allow you to move your forearms up and down. 3. Inhale and slowly lower the weights to the starting position. Do not allow yourself to rock back and forth and use momentum to lift the weights. Keep your wrists rigid throughout the movement. 4. Repeat 8–12 times.

This exercise can also be done with an exercise band. Stand on the band and hold the handles in your hands.

Exercise 17: One-Arm Extension with Weight   Level **II**

Casting a Fishing Line

PURPOSE
To increase upper arm strength for performing activities involving pushing motions (such as pushing up off a chair), improve range of motion, and create symmetry with the biceps.

MAIN MUSCLES WORKED
Back of upper arms (triceps).

STARTING POSITION A

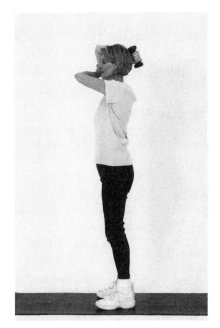

• Stand up straight
• Arms at your sides
• Feet shoulder width apart
• Knees slightly bent
• Abdominals contracted
• Lower back muscles contracted
• Shoulders down and back
• Chest lifted
• Look straight ahead

DESCRIPTION OF EXERCISE
1. Hold a weight in your right hand, raise your right arm above your head, and bend your right elbow so that it points straight up to the ceiling and your hand rests behind your head. **2.** Support your right arm with your left hand. **3.** Holding the left arm still, pull your shoulder blades down and back and hold them there. Exhale and straighten your right arm overhead. Do not rock or sway as you perform the movement. Do not lock your elbow. **4.** Inhale and bend your elbow back to the starting position. **5.** Perform 8–12 repetitions. **6.** Repeat on the other side.

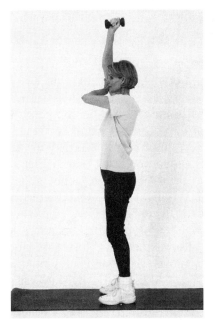

Level
II

Rolling Dough

PURPOSE
To increase strength of the forearms (grip strength). This exercise can help with everyday activities such as opening a tight jar or bottle top.

MAIN MUSCLES WORKED
Forearms (wrist flexors and extensors).

STARTING POSITION A

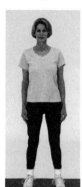

- Stand up straight
- Arms at your sides
- Feet shoulder width apart
- Knees slightly bent
- Abdominals contracted
- Lower back muscles contracted
- Shoulders down and back
- Chest lifted
- Look straight ahead

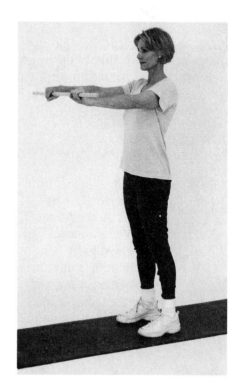

DESCRIPTION OF EXERCISE
1. Hold a dowel, with your arms shoulder width apart and your palms facing the floor. Raise the dowel, and straighten your arms out in front of you, keeping your elbows slightly bent. Hold your arms slightly above your heart or higher. This may be difficult but will encourage the flow of lymph. If it is too difficult, however, bend your elbows at a 90-degree angle so that your forearm is parallel to the floor. **2.** Rotate the dowel forward by bending your wrists, your hands moving toward the floor, 8–12 times. **3.** Reverse the wrist/hand movement to rotate the dowel backward in your hands 8–12 times. Do not exaggerate bending your wrist to perform the motion. Be sure to hold your arms and torso stationary and your shoulder blades down and back. Do not rock or sway as you perform the movement. Make sure that you are breathing consistently throughout the exercise. Don't hold your breath.

Exercise 19: Lower Back (Floor Work)

Modified Superwoman

PURPOSE
To strengthen the lower back and develop core body strength. This exercise is particularly beneficial for those who have had a TRAM flap. With any of the back exercises, stop if you feel any pain.

MAIN MUSCLES WORKED
Lower back (erector spinae), back of thighs (hamstrings), and buttocks (gluteals).

STARTING POSITION C

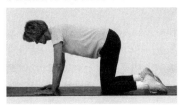

- On hands and knees
- Hands directly beneath shoulders (fingers face forward)
- Arms straight but not locked
- Knees shoulder width apart
- Head and neck a natural extension of the spine

DESCRIPTION OF EXERCISE
1. Raise your right arm straight out in front of you, no higher than shoulder level, and your left leg straight out behind you, no higher than hip level. Your body should be parallel to the floor. Squeeze your buttocks and contract your abdominals. Keep your head aligned with your spine, looking straight down. **2.** Hold the position for 5 seconds. **3.** Relax your buttocks and abdominals as you lower your arm and leg. **4.** Repeat the entire exercise with your left arm and right leg. **5.** Repeat steps 1–4, 6 times.

Remember to breathe consistently throughout the exercise. Do not hold your breath.

If you have any pain on your affected side, do not do this exercise but move on to Exercise 20.

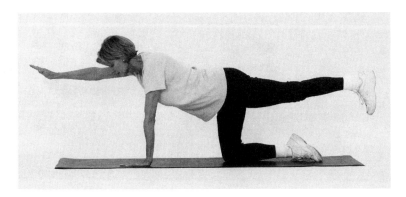

Exercise 20: Lower Back (Floor Work)

Superwoman

PURPOSE

To strengthen the lower back and develop core body strength. This exercise is particularly beneficial for those who have had a TRAM flap. With any of these back exercises, stop if you feel any pain.

MAIN MUSCLES WORKED

Lower back (erector spinae), back of thighs (hamstrings), and buttocks (gluteals).

STARTING POSITION

See "Description of Exercise."

DESCRIPTION OF EXERCISE

1. Lie facedown on the floor with your arms straight out in front of you. You may place a pillow or rolled-up towel under your forehead to keep your head and neck aligned with your spine. 2. Contract your abdominals and squeeze your buttocks. 3. Raise your right arm and left leg off the floor. Your head and chest will come up off the floor, but you will continue to look down, keeping your head and neck aligned with your spine. 4. Hold for 5 seconds. 5. Lower your arm and leg. 6. Repeat with your left arm and right leg. 7. Repeat steps 2–6, 8–12 times.

If needed, you can place a pillow under your chest and stomach or raise yourself up on one arm.

Remember to breathe consistently throughout the exercise. Do not hold your breath.

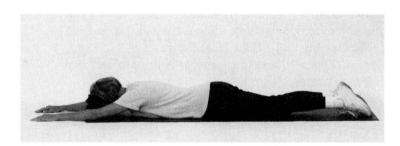

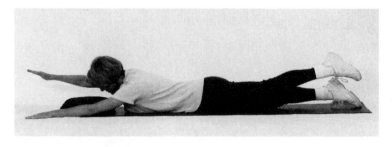

Exercise 21: Lower Back (Floor Work)

Bridging

PURPOSE
To strengthen the lower back and develop core body strength. This exercise is particularly beneficial for those who have had a TRAM flap. With any of the back exercises, stop if you feel any pain.

MAIN MUSCLES WORKED
Lower back (erector spinae), back of thighs (hamstrings), and buttocks (gluteals).

STARTING POSITION B

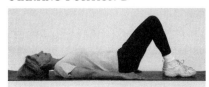

- Lie on your back
- Knees bent
- Feet flat on floor, hip width apart
- Abdominals contracted
- Small of your back pressed into the floor
- Arms straight at your sides, palms down

DESCRIPTION OF EXERCISE
1. Raise your hips (pelvis) off the floor by contracting your abdominals, lower back, and buttocks until your body forms a straight line from your kneecaps and thighs to your chin. Be sure to keep your shoulders and upper back in contact with the floor. **2.** Keeping your pelvis level, hold the straight-line position for 5 seconds. **3.** Lower your hips back to the floor. **4.** Repeat 8–12 times.

Remember to breathe consistently throughout the exercise. Do not hold your breath.

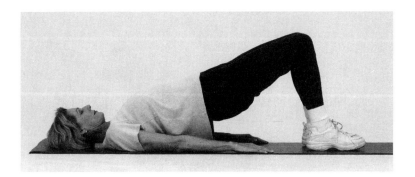

Exercise 22: Abdominals (Floor Work)

Bending in Half

PURPOSE
To strengthen the abdominals and provide core body strength. This exercise may be contraindicated for those who have had a TRAM flap. The exercise will help improve posture, which can be adversely affected by mastectomy and reconstructive surgery.

MAIN MUSCLES WORKED
Abdominals (rectus abdominis, transverse abdominis, obliques).

STARTING POSITION B

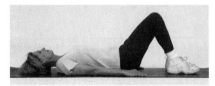

- Lie on your back
- Knees bent
- Feet flat on floor, hip width apart
- Abdominals contracted
- Small of your back pressed into the floor
- Arms straight at your sides, palms down

DESCRIPTION OF EXERCISE/PELVIC TILT
1. Flatten your lower back into the floor by contracting your abdominals and buttocks at the same time. If you have trouble with the motion, think of pressing the small of your back into the floor as if you were trying to squish a grape between your lower back and the floor. **2.** Hold the position for 5 seconds and then return to the starting position. **3.** Repeat 8–12 times.

This exercise can also be done with your legs straight or while standing (place your back against a wall if you need support while doing this exercise in a standing position).

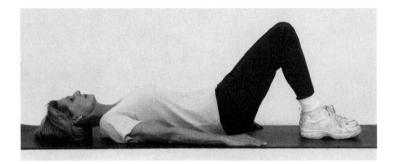

DESCRIPTION OF EXERCISE/BASIC CRUNCH

1. Tilt your pelvis so that your lower back is flat on the floor. Keeping your arms extended at your sides, slowly lift your shoulders and head off the floor using your abdominals (think of pulling your navel toward the floor). Keep your chin in a steady position (as if you were holding someone's fist in place under your chin—do not let your head fall back or tuck your chin to your chest). Do not come up so far that your lower back comes off the floor. **2.** Pause briefly. **3.** Lower yourself slowly. **4.** Repeat 8–12 times.

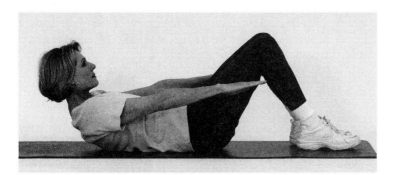

DESCRIPTION OF EXERCISE/OBLIQUE WORK

1. Perform the same exercise as the Basic Crunch but add a slight twist. As you keep your arms extended and lift your shoulders and head off the floor, reach with both hands to the outside of your right leg. **2.** Pause. **3.** Lower yourself slowly back to the floor. **4.** Perform the lift 8–12 times. **5.** Repeat the lift, reaching to the outside of the left leg.

Remember to breathe consistently throughout the exercises. Do not hold your breath. You may find it helpful to exhale as you raise yourself up and inhale as you lower yourself back down. You want to make sure that you pull your navel toward your spine as you perform the exercise. Don't let your stomach "puff out."

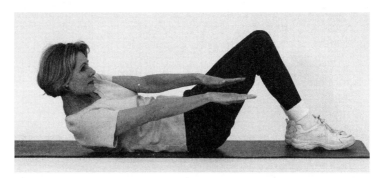

Exercise 23: Abdominals (Standing)

Cheerleader

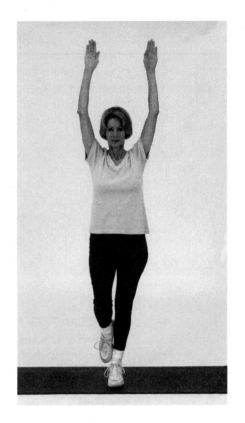

PURPOSE
To strengthen the abdominals and provide core body strength. This exercise may not be appropriate for those who have had a TRAM flap. The exercise will help improve posture, which can be adversely affected by mastectomy and reconstructive surgery.

MAIN MUSCLES WORKED
Abdominals (rectus abdominis, transverse abdominis, obliques).

STARTING POSITION A

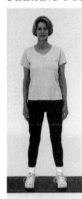

- Stand up straight
- Arms at your sides
- Feet shoulder width apart
- Knees slightly bent
- Abdominals contracted
- Lower back muscles contracted
- Shoulders down and back
- Chest lifted
- Look straight ahead

DESCRIPTION OF EXERCISE
1. Stand on one leg and hold the other leg so that your toes are resting next to the ankle of the standing leg. Contract your abdominals and buttocks to stabilize your torso. **2.** Slowly flap your arms out to the sides and up over your head like a bird in flight 8–12 times. **3.** Bring your arms to your sides, with your palms against the sides of your legs. **4.** Move your arms up and down in front of you in a scissorslike motion 8–12 times. **5.** Hold your arms

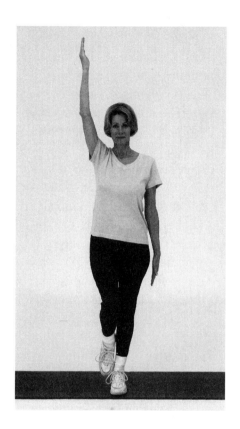

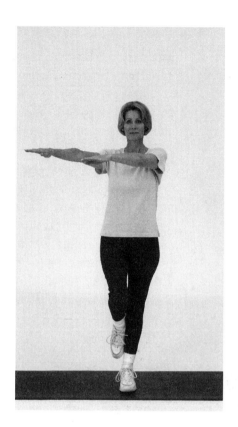

straight out in front of you at shoulder height, with your palms facing the floor. **6.** Keeping your elbows straight, move your arms together from side to side in front of you, without letting your shoulders or torso move (the only motion is at the shoulder joint), 8–12 times. **7.** Repeat steps 2–6 while standing on your other leg.

Keep breathing regularly throughout the exercise. Move your arms in a controlled manner in all steps of this exercise.

Level III

Level III follows the same principles as Level II but incorporates different exercises and a higher intensity level. In Level III, you will increase the amount of resistance you use and, in some cases, the number of repetitions you perform. Several "combination exercises" are included, in which you perform two different exercises together to complete one repetition.

You may progress from Level III to Level IV when you have achieved two to three sets of 8–12 repetitions of each exercise. Do not progress if you do not feel up to it. If you experience pain or loss of range of motion, stop exercising and see your doctor.

Remember, your arm's response to exercise is your ultimate indicator for progressing in your program. If you feel pain or notice redness, change in skin texture, or swelling, stop exercising and call your doctor immediately. If you are given the OK to continue, reduce the number of repetitions and the resistance you are using. You may want to go back to the previous level.

Take a moment to review "Points to Remember When Performing All Exercises" on page 46. Don't forget that your progression should be very gradual. Listen to your body and create your own plan for living stronger.

Level III Exercises

	TECHNICAL NAME	ANALOGY NAME
Exercise 1	Bent-Over Row	Starting the Lawn Mower
Exercise 2	Lunge	Ballet Skiing
Exercise 3	Modified Floor Push-ups Followed by Chest Flies	Looking for Lost Contact Lens/Hugging a Barrel
Exercise 4	Supine Leg Lifts with Ankle Weights	Traction
Exercise 5	Low Row with Band	Pulling on a Horse's Reins
Exercise 6	Exercise Ball Squat with Lateral Raise	Jumping Jacks
Exercise 7	Shoulder Blade Squeeze with Band	Advanced Chicken Wings
Exercise 8	Hamstring Curls with Weights	Advanced Balancing Act
Exercise 9	Lying Pull Over and Serratus Reach with Weights	Playing with a Baby
Exercise 10	Standing Knee Raise with Leg Extension	Cancan Girl
Exercise 11	Front-to-Back Reach	Skiing Moguls

Exercise 12	Plié with Calf Raise Using Weights	Clumsy Ballerina
Exercise 13	Internal Rotation (Shoulder/Rotator Cuff)	Pulling the Door Shut
Exercise 14	External Rotation (Shoulder/Rotator Cuff)	Opening the Door
Exercise 15	Biceps Curl with Weights or Band	Popeye Showing Off for Olive Oyl
Exercise 16	One-Arm Extension with Weight	Casting a Fishing Line
Exercise 17	Reverse Curls with Dowel or Weights	Lifting the Security Bar on a Carnival Ride
Exercise 18	Ball or Towel Squeeze	Kneading Dough
Exercise 19	Lower Back (Floor Work)	Modified Superwoman
Exercise 20	Lower Back (Floor Work)	Superwoman
Exercise 21	Lower Back (Floor Work)	Bridging
Exercise 22	Abdominals (Floor Work)	Bending in Half
Exercise 23	Abdominals (Standing)	Cheerleader

Level

III

Starting the Lawn Mower

PURPOSE

To strengthen the back muscles while stretching the incision and skin across the chest wall. This will help alleviate the tightness of the chest muscles and strengthen weak back muscles, which can impair your posture by pulling the shoulder forward and giving you a hunchbacked appearance.

MAIN MUSCLES WORKED

Back (lower latissimus dorsi, middle trapezius, rhomboids) and back of shoulders (posterior deltoids).

STARTING POSITION A

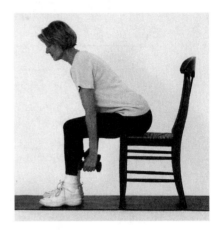

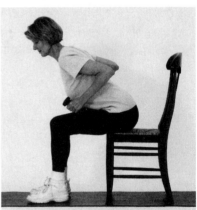

- Stand up straight
- Arms at your sides
- Feet shoulder width apart
- Knees slightly bent
- Abdominals contracted
- Lower back muscles contracted
- Shoulders down and back
- Chest lifted
- Look straight ahead

DESCRIPTION OF EXERCISE

1. Sitting on the edge of a chair, bend forward from your hips and support your torso on your thighs. Keep your back straight and your head and neck aligned with your spine. Holding a 1- to 5-pound weight in each hand, let your arms hang straight down from your shoulders with your palms facing in. **2.** Keeping your shoulders down and your abdominals contracted, exhale as you pull the weights up to your hips, leading with your elbows. Your shoulder blades will move toward your spine. Keep your elbows pointing behind you—not out to your side. Do not rock or sway as you perform the movement. Keep control of the weights throughout the movement. **3.** Pause for a second. **4.** Inhale and slowly lower the weights back down to the starting position, keeping your shoulder blades anchored against your spine. **5.** Relax your shoulder blades. **6.** Repeat 8–12 times.

Exercise 2: Lunge

Ballet Skiing

PURPOSE

To improve posture and balance, strengthen and stabilize the torso, and improve lower body strength and range of motion. Stabilizing your torso will help protect your lower back from injury and strengthen the muscles used in everyday activities such as sitting, standing, and walking.

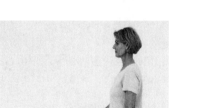

MAIN MUSCLES WORKED

Buttocks (gluteals), back of thighs (hamstrings) and front of thighs (quadriceps).

STARTING POSITION A

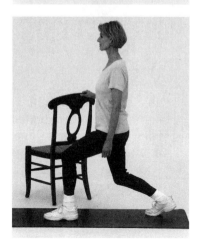

- Stand up straight
- Arms at your sides
- Feet shoulder width apart
- Knees slightly bent
- Abdominals contracted
- Lower back muscles contracted
- Shoulders down and back
- Chest lifted
- Look straight ahead

DESCRIPTION OF EXERCISE

1. Stand next to a chair. Take a step forward with your left foot so that it is 2–3 feet in front of the right, and your feet are hip width apart. Your hips should be directly under your shoulders and your torso upright. Your arms hang by your sides or rest on your hips. **2.** Bend both knees so that your left knee is over your left ankle, your left lower leg is perpendicular to the floor, your right lower leg is parallel to the floor, and your right heel is lifted. Both legs should be bent at 90 degrees. (If they are not, adjust the position of your feet.) Keep your abdominals contracted, your rib cage lifted, and your torso upright. **3.** Squeeze your buttocks and straighten both legs to raise yourself back up to the step 1 position. **4.** Repeat 8–12 times. **5.** Repeat steps 1–4 with your right foot forward. Keep breathing!

If 90 degrees is too difficult for you, start by lowering yourself a quarter of the way down.

Level
III

Looking for Lost Contact Lens/Hugging a Barrel

PURPOSE

To strengthen the muscles of the chest wall and improve upper body range of motion.

MAIN MUSCLES WORKED

Chest (pectorals), front of shoulders (anterior deltoids), back of upper arms (triceps), and a shoulder girdle muscle (serratus anterior).

STARTING POSITION C

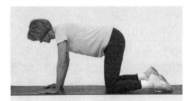

- On hands and knees
- Hands directly beneath shoulders (fingers face forward)
- Arms straight but not locked
- Knees shoulder width apart
- Head and neck a natural extension of the spine

DESCRIPTION OF EXERCISE

1. Get on the floor on your hands and knees. Keep your head aligned with your spine, your abdominals contracted, and your back flat throughout the exercise. **2.** Inhale as you lower yourself toward the floor to within 3–5 inches of the floor (or as far as is comfortable), by bending your elbows. Be sure to contract your abdominals and squeeze your buttocks to stabilize your torso. Don't let your back droop. If you feel pain in your lower back, adjust your position. **3.** Contract your chest muscles (imagine squeezing a banana under each armpit) and push yourself away from the floor by straightening your elbows (be sure not to lock them). **4.** Repeat 8–12 times.

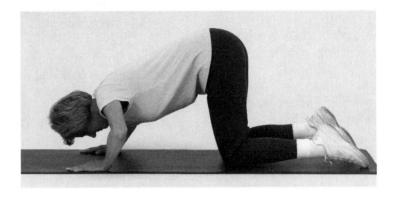

5. Turn over and lie on your back, with your knees bent and your feet flat. Hold a 1- to 5-pound weight in each hand. Raise your hands straight up in the air above your chest, with your palms facing each other. Contract your chest, feeling the tension in your armpits. **6.** Keeping a slight bend in your elbows, slowly lower your arms out to the sides as far as is comfortable (pretend you are holding a barrel in your arms). **7.** Contract your chest, feeling the tension in your armpits, then bring your arms back up above your chest. **8.** Repeat 8–12 times.

If you feel any pain in your arm or chest with either exercise, stop the exercise and return to a lower level chest exercise.

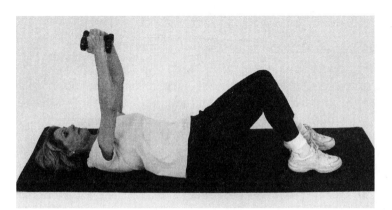

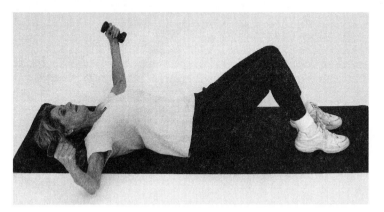

Level
III

Exercise 4: Supine Leg Lifts with Ankle Weights

Traction

PURPOSE
To strengthen legs and hip flexors, which are involved in everyday movements such as sitting, standing, and walking.

MAIN MUSCLES WORKED
Front of thighs (quadriceps), hip flexors, abdominals, and lower back (erector spinae).

STARTING POSITION D

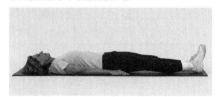

- Lie on your back
- Legs straight
- Arms straight at your sides, palms down

DESCRIPTION OF EXERCISE
1. Wear a 1- to 2-pound ankle weight on each leg. Contract your abdominals and press the small of your back against the floor (pelvic tilt). Keep your back in contact with the floor throughout the exercise. Bend your right knee and place your right foot flat on the floor. Keep your left leg straight. **2.** Keeping your left foot flexed, raise your left leg as high as you can, but no higher than 45 degrees. **3.** Pause. **4.** Slowly lower your left leg until it is about an inch above the floor. **5.** Repeat the lift 8–12 times. **6.** Repeat steps 2–5 with the right leg.

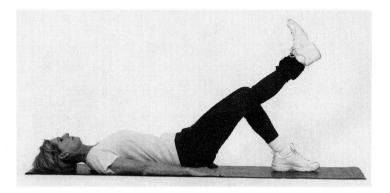

Exercise 5: Low Row with Band   Level

III

Pulling on a Horse's Reins

PURPOSE
To strengthen upper back and shoulder girdle muscles, improve muscle symmetry, promote muscle awareness, increase upper body range of motion, and improve posture.

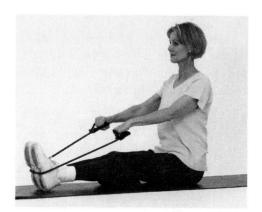

MAIN MUSCLES WORKED
Back (latissimus dorsi, rhomboids, trapezius), back of shoulders (posterior deltoids), and front of upper arms (biceps).

STARTING POSITION
See "Description of Exercise."

DESCRIPTION OF EXERCISE
1. Sit on the floor with your legs straight out in front of you. Grasp the end of an exercise band in each hand and put the middle of the band under the soles of your feet. **2.** Extend your arms straight out in front of you, with your palms facing down. Make sure the band is secure around your feet and stretched taut with low tension. (You should not feel pain holding the band.) Contract your abdominals and sit upright, lifting your rib cage, pulling your shoulder blades down and back, and looking straight ahead. **3.** Exhale as you pull your elbows back as if you could touch them behind you. Keep your elbows raised to just below shoulder level. Don't shrug your shoulders, and keep your torso perfectly still. Keep your abdominals contracted. **4.** Pause, squeezing your shoulder blades together. **5.** Inhale as you return your arms to the starting position. **6.** Repeat 8–12 times.

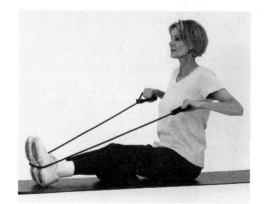

Level

III

Jumping Jacks

PURPOSE

To improve posture by promoting muscle strength and awareness, strengthen the lower body and shoulders, and improve stabilization of the body core.

MAIN MUSCLES WORKED

Buttocks (gluteals), front of thighs (quadriceps), back of thighs (hamstrings), shoulders (deltoids), and a rotator cuff muscle (supraspinatus).

STARTING POSITION A

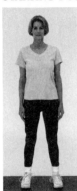

- Stand up straight
- Arms at your sides
- Feet shoulder width apart
- Knees slightly bent
- Abdominals contracted
- Lower back muscles contracted
- Shoulders down and back
- Chest lifted
- Look straight ahead

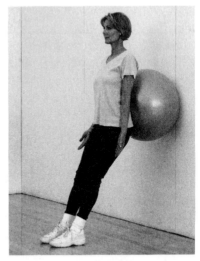

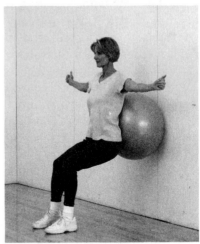

DESCRIPTION OF EXERCISE

1. Stand near the wall with an exercise ball in the small of your back and against the wall. Walk your legs out about 18 inches, keeping your feet shoulder width apart and your toes pointing forward. Your arms should hang by your sides, with your palms facing your thighs. **2.** Inhale as you press back firmly against the ball and lower your torso by bending your knees while raising your arms out to the side to shoulder height. Squeeze your shoulder blades down and back and hold them there before you raise your arms. Your palms will face the floor. Go as low as you comfortably can, but no lower than with your knees bent at a 90-degree angle. **3.** Exhale as you straighten your legs and lower your arms back to your sides. Do not lock your knees or elbows. Keep your head and neck straight and look forward. **4.** Repeat 8–12 times.

If it feels more natural for you, breathe in the opposite pattern from that described above.

Exercise 7: Shoulder Blade Squeeze with Band

Advanced Chicken Wings

PURPOSE

To improve posture by increasing muscular awareness, strengthening the upper back, and reducing any forward rounding of the back (kyphosis).

MAIN MUSCLES WORKED

Upper back (rhomboids), mid-back (middle and lower trapezius), back of shoulders (posterior deltoids), and a rotator cuff muscle (teres minor).

STARTING POSITION A

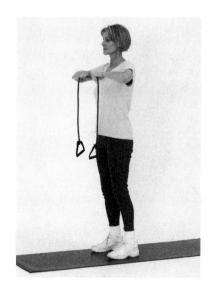

• Stand up straight
• Arms at your sides
• Feet shoulder width apart
• Knees slightly bent
• Abdominals contracted
• Lower back muscles contracted
• Shoulders down and back
• Chest lifted
• Look straight ahead

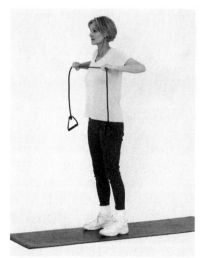

DESCRIPTION OF EXERCISE

1. Hold an exercise band with your hands about shoulder width apart (closer together for more tension). Raise your arms to shoulder height or just below and bend your elbows so that your fingertips are touching in front of your chest. Your arms stay parallel to the ground. Keep your palms facing down. **2.** Pull your shoulder blades down and back (together) and hold them there as you draw your elbows back as if you could touch them behind you. Keep your arms at the same height as your starting position as you move your elbows back. Do not shrug your shoulders up toward your ears. If the tension on the band is too great, place your hands farther apart on the band. The tension should be low and not cause any pain. **3.** Hold for 5 seconds. **4.** Bring your elbows back toward the front so that your fingertips are touching as in the starting position. Release your shoulder blades. **5.** Repeat steps 2–4, 8–12 times.

Level III

Exercise 8: Hamstring Curls with Weights

Advanced Balancing Act

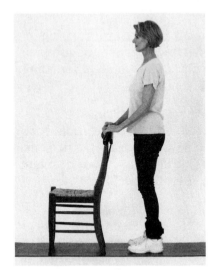

PURPOSE

To improve posture and balance and increase leg strength, which is vital to performing everyday activities and maintaining functional independence.

MAIN MUSCLES WORKED

Back of thighs (hamstrings).

STARTING POSITION F

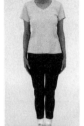

- Stand up straight
- Arms at your sides
- Feet together
- Knees slightly bent
- Abdominals contracted
- Lower back muscles contracted
- Shoulders down and back
- Chest lifted
- Look straight ahead

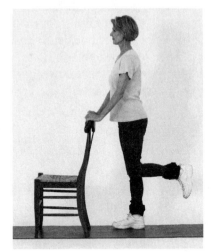

DESCRIPTION OF EXERCISE

1. Wear a 1- to 2-pound ankle weight on each leg. Hold on to the back of a chair for balance. (If you used weights in Level II, Exercise 8, try to increase your resistance.) **2.** Keeping your thighs parallel, exhale and bend one knee, lifting the heel toward the buttocks. The heel does not need to come any closer than 45 degrees from the buttocks. Keep your foot flexed throughout the motion (don't point your toes). Keep the knee of the bent leg centered underneath the hip, next to the stationary knee. (If the thigh moves backward you may place undue stress on the knee.) Focus on the muscle contraction in the back of the upper leg as you bend the knee. Only the knee joint is moving. Throughout the exercise, contract your abdominals and buttocks, keep your pelvis level and still, lift your rib cage, look straight ahead, keep the knee of your support leg slightly bent, keep your foot flexed, and keep your torso straight and upright (do not bend at the hips or waist). **3.** Inhale and slowly straighten your knee and return to the starting position. **4.** Repeat 8–12 times. **5.** Repeat the exercise with the other leg.

Exercise 9: Lying Pull Over and Serratus Reach with Weights

Playing with a Baby/ Reaching for the Stars

PURPOSE
To improve torso stability, increase muscle symmetry, increase upper body range of motion, and strengthen shoulder girdle muscles. This exercise also will help prevent feelings of weakness in the arm when reaching in front of you.

MAIN MUSCLES WORKED
Back (latissimus dorsi), upper back (rhomboids), chest (pectorals), and a shoulder girdle muscle (serratus anterior).

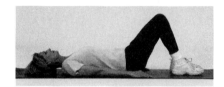

STARTING POSITION B
- Lie on your back
- Knees bent
- Feet flat on floor, hip width apart
- Abdominals contracted
- Small of your back pressed into the floor
- Arms straight at your sides, palms down

DESCRIPTION OF EXERCISE
1. Hold a 1- to 5-pound weight in each hand and extend your arms toward the ceiling above your chest. (You may also hold one weight with both hands, as shown in the photograph.) Pull your shoulder blades down and back (together) and hold them there. **2.** Inhale deeply as you lower your arms over your head toward the floor until you feel a mild stretch in your chest and armpit (axilla). Keep your arms straight (but with a slight bend in the elbows), your buttocks and lower back pressed down into the floor, and your upper arms close to your head. **3.** Exhale as you pull your shoulder blades down and back, contract your chest muscles, and raise your arms back to the starting position. Focus on your back and chest muscles to perform the movement. **4.** Take a deep breath, then exhale as you reach for the ceiling by raising your arms as high as you can, lifting your shoulders off the floor and keeping your elbows straight but not locked (your head and upper back stay on the floor). Keep your abdominals contracted, your torso still, your lower back flat on the floor, and your shoulder blades anchored down and back throughout the movement (see photo on page 162). Focus on stability. **5.** Hold your arms up for 5 seconds, breathing normally. **6.** Inhale as you lower your arms back to the starting position. **7.** Repeat steps 2–6, 8–12 times.

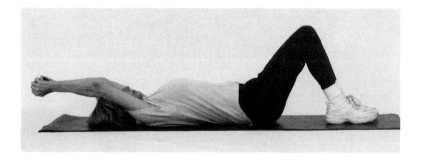

Level

III

Cancan Girl

PURPOSE
To increase torso stability, improve posture, and increase hip flexor strength. This exercise, particularly the flexion in the hips during the knee raise, may be difficult if you have had a TRAM flap.

MAIN MUSCLES WORKED
Hip flexors and front of thighs (quadriceps).

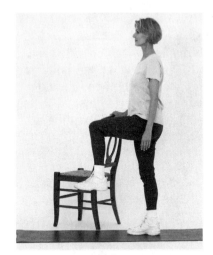

STARTING POSITION A

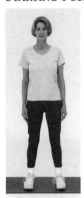

- Stand up straight
- Arms at your sides
- Feet shoulder width apart
- Knees slightly bent
- Abdominals contracted
- Lower back muscles contracted
- Shoulders down and back
- Chest lifted
- Look straight ahead

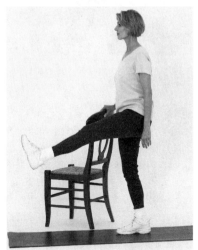

DESCRIPTION OF EXERCISE
1. Stand next to a chair for balance.
2. Exhale and bend one knee at a 90-degree angle in front of you as if lifting the upper thigh toward your abdomen. The knee of the moving leg does not need to come higher than hip level. Keep your pelvis level and still. 3. Inhale then exhale as you slowly straighten your leg out in front of you as if you were kicking a ball. Extend your leg as far as you can, keeping your back straight, but don't lock your knee. 4. Inhale and slowly bend the knee and lower your leg to the starting position, with both feet flat on the floor. 5. Repeat 8–12 times. 6. Move the chair to your right side for support and repeat steps 2–5.

For added resistance, you can wear 1- to 2-pound ankle weights while performing this exercise.

Throughout the exercise, contract your abdominals and buttocks, lift your rib cage, look straight ahead, and keep your torso straight and upright (do not bend at the hips or waist).

Exercise 11: Front-to-Back Reach

Skiing Moguls

PURPOSE
To increase shoulder range of motion, upper body strength and symmetry, and torso stability.

MAIN MUSCLES WORKED
Shoulders (deltoids), chest (pectorals), and back (rhomboids, latissimus dorsi, lower trapezius).

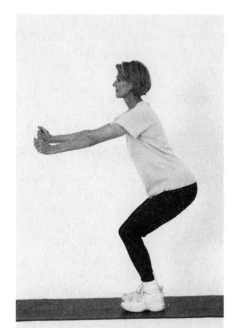

STARTING POSITION A

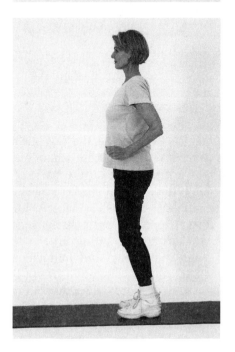

- Stand up straight
- Arms at your sides
- Feet shoulder width apart
- Knees slightly bent
- Abdominals contracted
- Lower back muscles contracted
- Shoulders down and back
- Chest lifted
- Look straight ahead

DESCRIPTION OF EXERCISE
1. Inhale as you bend slightly forward from your hips and squat back as if you were going to sit in a chair (keeping the natural arch to your back and making sure your knees stay behind your toes). Raise your arms out in front of you, with your palms facing down. Your hands should be at about eye level and your elbows only slightly bent. **2.** Exhale as you straighten your legs, keeping your knees slightly bent, and bring your hips slightly forward into a pelvic thrust, while lowering your arms and pulling them in to your sides. **3.** Perform 8–12 repetitions.

Level III

Exercise 12: Plié with Calf Raise Using Weights

Clumsy Ballerina

PURPOSE:
To improve balance by strengthening the ankle and foot, improve stability, and strengthen the legs.

MAIN MUSCLES WORKED
Buttocks (gluteals), front of thighs (quadriceps), some inner thighs (adductors), and back of calves (gastrocnemius and soleus).

STARTING POSITION E

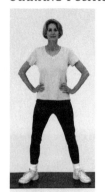

- Stand up straight
- Hands on hips
- Feet wider than shoulder width apart
- Toes turned out slightly to the side
- Knees slightly bent
- Abdominals contracted
- Lower back muscles contracted
- Shoulders down and back
- Chest lifted
- Look straight ahead

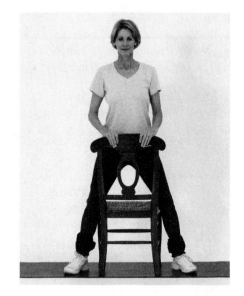

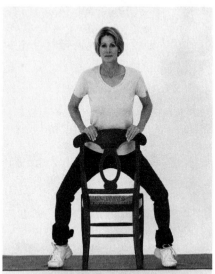

DESCRIPTION OF EXERCISE
1. Wear a 1- to 5-pound ankle weight on each leg. **2.** Assume the starting position, with your legs straddling the seat of a chair and your arms resting on the back of the chair for support. **3.** Inhale as you raise up on the balls of your feet, bend your knees, and lower your buttocks straight down until you are almost sitting on the chair. Keep your abdominals and buttocks contracted and your back straight. Don't bend forward or backward and don't let your knees travel past your toes. **4.** Exhale as you straighten your legs, squeezing your buttocks as you raise yourself to the starting position and lower your heels to the floor. **5.** Repeat steps 3 and 4, 8–12 times.

Exercise 13: Internal Rotation (Shoulder/Rotator Cuff)

Pulling the Door Shut

PURPOSE

To increase range of motion in shoulder rotation, strengthen the rotator cuff, and improve stability of the shoulder joint.

MAIN MUSCLES WORKED

Chest (pectoralis major), back (latissimus dorsi and teres major), rotator cuff (subscapularis), and front of shoulders (anterior deltoids).

STARTING POSITION

See "Description of Exercise."

DESCRIPTION OF EXERCISE

1. Lie on your right side on the floor and bend your knees so that they are in front of you to provide support. Keep your left knee on top of your right. Place a pillow (or equivalent) under your head so that your head stays aligned with your spine. Rest your left arm on your side. **2.** Stretch your right arm straight out on the floor in front of you, palm toward the ceiling, and bend the elbow at a 90-degree angle to bring your upper arm back next to your side, with your elbow near your waist. (Keep your arm on the floor.) Hold a 1- to 5-pound weight in your right hand. (Try to increase your resistance from Level II, Exercise 13.) **3.** Exhale and rotate your forearm toward the ceiling, leading with the palm. Keep your upper arm on the floor. Keep your wrist straight. **4.** Inhale and return to the starting position. **5.** Repeat 8–12 times. **6.** Repeat on the other side.

If you choose to use a weight, as shown in the photograph, begin with 1 to 2 pounds.

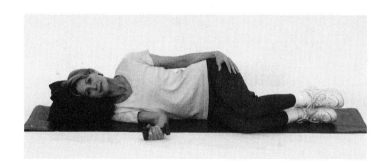

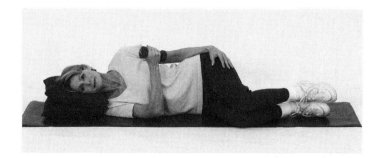

Exercise 14: External Rotation (Shoulder/Rotator Cuff)

Opening the Door

PURPOSE
To increase range of motion in shoulder rotation, strengthen the rotator cuff, and improve stability of the shoulder joint.

MAIN MUSCLES WORKED
Rotator cuff (infraspinatus and teres minor) and back of the shoulder (posterior deltoid).

STARTING POSITION
See "Description of Exercise."

DESCRIPTION OF EXERCISE
1. Lie on your right side on the floor and bend your knees so that they are in front of you to provide support. Keep your left knee on top of your right. Support your head with your right arm. 2. Hold a 1- to 5-pound weight in your left hand. Bend the elbow of your left arm at a 90-degree angle and rest your elbow on your hip. Your forearm should be parallel to the floor and your hand (holding the weight) palm down. 3. Exhale and rotate your forearm toward the ceiling, leading with the back of your hand. Your elbow stays on your hip, and your upper arm stays by your side. Keep your wrist straight. 4. Inhale and return to the starting position. 5. Repeat 8–12 times. 6. Repeat on the other side.

If you choose to use a weight, as shown in the photograph, begin with 1 to 2 pounds.

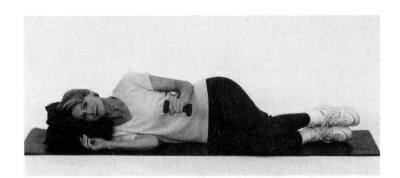

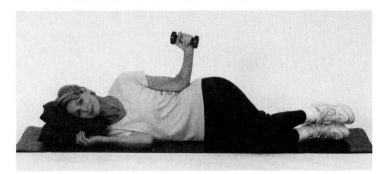

Exercise 15: Biceps Curl with Weights or Band   Level

Popeye Showing Off for Olive Oyl

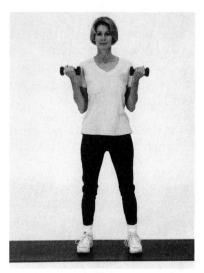

PURPOSE
To increase upper arm strength for performing everyday activities involving pulling motions.

MAIN MUSCLES WORKED
Front of upper arms (biceps).

STARTING POSITION A

- Stand up straight
- Arms at your sides
- Feet shoulder width apart
- Knees slightly bent
- Abdominals contracted
- Lower back muscles contracted
- Shoulders down and back
- Chest lifted
- Look straight ahead

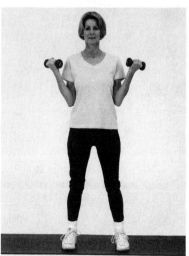

DESCRIPTION OF EXERCISE
1. Hold a 1- to 5-pound weight in each hand and hang your arms straight down at your sides, with your palms facing forward. Keep your elbows close by your sides and directly under your shoulders. Keep your shoulder blades down and back throughout the movement. **2.** Bend your elbows and exhale as you curl your forearms toward your shoulders. Imagine your elbows as pivot points that allow you to move your forearms up and down. Keep your wrists rigid and press your upper arms into your body as you lift, as if holding a newspaper under your arm. Do not allow yourself to rock back and forth and use momentum to lift the weights. **3.** Inhale as you lower your forearms slowly to the starting position. **4.** Turn your arms so that your palms are angled away from your body. **5.** Perform steps 2 and 3 with your arms in this position. **6.** Repeat steps 1–5, 8–12 times.

This exercise can also be done with an exercise band. Stand on the band and hold the handles in your hands.

Level

III

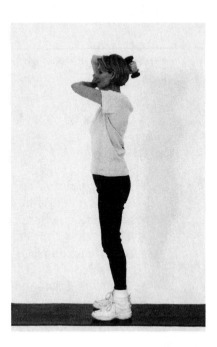

Exercise 16: One-Arm Extension with Weight

Casting a Fishing Line

PURPOSE

To increase upper arm strength for performing activities involving pushing motions (such as pushing up off a chair), improve range of motion, and create symmetry with the biceps.

MAIN MUSCLES WORKED

Back of upper arms (triceps).

STARTING POSITION A

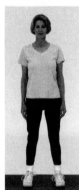

- Stand up straight
- Arms at your sides
- Feet shoulder width apart
- Knees slightly bent
- Abdominals contracted
- Lower back muscles contracted
- Shoulders down and back
- Chest lifted
- Look straight ahead

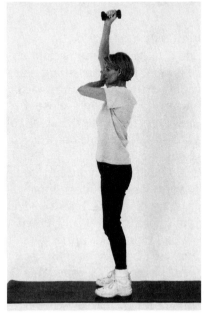

DESCRIPTION OF EXERCISE

1. Hold a weight in your right hand, raise your right arm above your head, and bend your right elbow so that it points straight up to the ceiling and your hand rests behind your head. **2.** Support your right arm with your left hand. **3.** Holding the left arm still, pull your shoulder blades down and back and hold them there. Exhale and straighten your right arm overhead. Do not rock or sway as you perform the movement. Do not lock your elbow. **4.** Inhale and bend your elbow back to the starting position. **5.** Perform 8–12 repetitions. **6.** Repeat on the other side.

Exercise 17: Reverse Curls with Dowel or Weights

Lifting the Security Bar on a Carnival Ride

PURPOSE
To increase the strength of the elbow flexors.

MAIN MUSCLES WORKED
Elbow flexors (brachioradialis) and wrist extensors.

STARTING POSITION A

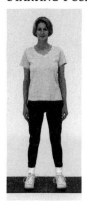

- Stand up straight
- Arms at your sides
- Feet shoulder width apart
- Knees slightly bent
- Abdominals contracted
- Lower back muscles contracted
- Shoulders down and back
- Chest lifted
- Look straight ahead

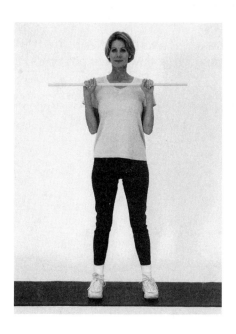

DESCRIPTION OF EXERCISE
1. Bend your arms so that your forearms are parallel to the floor. Hold a dowel, with your palms facing the floor and your hands approximately shoulder width apart. **2.** Keeping your upper arms close by your sides and your elbows directly under your shoulders, exhale as you bend your elbows and raise the dowel up toward your face as far as you can. Curl the back of your forearms toward your chest. Keep your wrists straight. **3.** Inhale as you slowly lower the dowel back to the starting position. **4.** Repeat 8–12 times.

For added resistance, instead hold a 1- to 5-pound weight in each hand.

Level

III

Exercise 18: Ball or Towel Squeeze

Kneading Dough

PURPOSE

To improve forearm and grip strength and to improve the flow of lymph.

MAIN MUSCLES WORKED

Forearms (wrist flexors, wrist extensors).

STARTING POSITION B

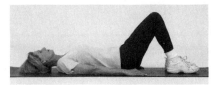

- Lie on your back
- Knees bent
- Feet flat on floor, hip width apart
- Abdominals contracted
- Small of your back pressed into the floor
- Arms straight at your sides, palms down

DESCRIPTION OF EXERCISE

1. Holding a "squeezable" ball (the size of a tennis ball or smaller) in each hand, raise your arms straight up toward the ceiling so that they are perpendicular to the floor. **2.** Squeeze the balls and release 8–12 times.

This exercise can also be done with a folded towel in each hand.

If you have nothing to hold, make a fist with each hand. Squeeze and then release.

Remember to breathe consistently throughout the exercise. Do not hold your breath.

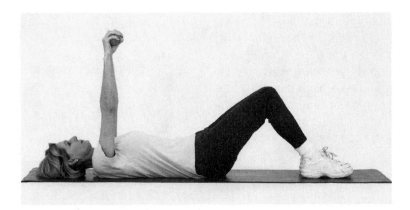

Exercise 19: Lower Back (Floor Work) | **Level III**

Modified Superwoman

PURPOSE

To strengthen the lower back and develop core body strength. This exercise is particularly beneficial for those who have had a TRAM flap. With any of the back exercises, stop if you feel any pain.

MAIN MUSCLES WORKED

Lower back (erector spinae), back of thighs (hamstrings), and buttocks (gluteals).

STARTING POSITION C

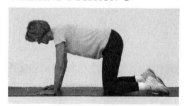

- On hands and knees
- Hands directly beneath shoulders (fingers face forward)
- Arms straight but not locked
- Knees shoulder width apart
- Head and neck a natural extension of the spine

DESCRIPTION OF EXERCISE

1. Raise your right arm straight out in front of you, no higher than shoulder level, and your left leg straight out behind you, no higher than hip level. Your body should be parallel to the floor. Squeeze your buttocks and contract your abdominals. Keep your head aligned with your spine, looking straight down. **2.** Hold the position for 5 seconds. **3.** Relax your buttocks and abdominals as you lower your arm and leg. **4.** Repeat the entire exercise with your left arm and right leg. **5.** Repeat steps 1–4, 6 times.

Remember to breathe consistently throughout the exercise. Do not hold your breath.

If you have any pain on your affected side, do not do this exercise but move on to Exercise 20.

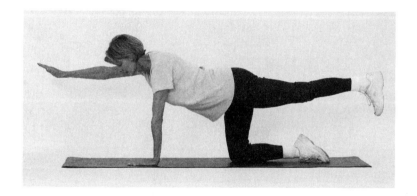

Exercise 20: Lower Back (Floor Work)

Superwoman

PURPOSE
To strengthen the lower back and develop core body strength. This exercise is particularly beneficial for those who have had a TRAM flap. With any of the back exercises, stop if you feel any pain.

MAIN MUSCLES WORKED
Lower back (erector spinae), back of thighs (hamstrings), and buttocks (gluteals).

STARTING POSITION
See "Description of Exercise."

DESCRIPTION OF EXERCISE
1. Lie facedown on the floor with your arms straight out in front of you. You may place a pillow or rolled-up towel under your forehead to keep your head and neck aligned with your spine. 2. Contract your abdominals and squeeze your buttocks. 3. Raise your right arm and left leg off the floor. Your head and chest will come up off the floor, but you will continue to look down, keeping your head and neck aligned with your spine. 4. Hold for 5 seconds. 5. Lower your arm and leg. 6. Repeat with your left arm and right leg. 7. Repeat steps 2–6, 8–12 times.

If needed, you can place a pillow under your chest and stomach or raise yourself up on one arm.

Remember to breathe consistently throughout the exercise. Do not hold your breath.

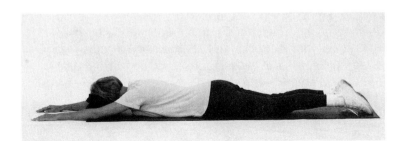

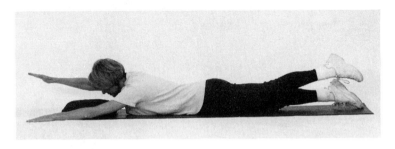

Exercise 21: Lower Back (Floor Work)

Bridging

PURPOSE

To strengthen the lower back and develop core body strength. This exercise is particularly beneficial for those who have had a TRAM flap. With any of the back exercises, stop if you feel any pain.

MAIN MUSCLES WORKED

Lower back (erector spinae), back of thighs (hamstrings), and buttocks (gluteals).

STARTING POSITION B

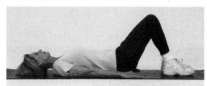

- Lie on your back
- Knees bent
- Feet flat on floor, hip width apart
- Abdominals contracted
- Small of your back pressed into the floor
- Arms straight at your sides, palms down

DESCRIPTION OF EXERCISE

1. Raise your hips (pelvis) off the floor by contracting your abdominals, lower back, and buttocks until your body forms a straight line from your kneecaps and thighs to your chin. Be sure to keep your shoulders and upper back in contact with the floor. **2.** Keeping your pelvis level, hold the straight-line position for 5 seconds. **3.** Lower your hips back to the floor. **4.** Repeat 8–12 times.

Remember to breathe consistently throughout the exercise. Do not hold your breath.

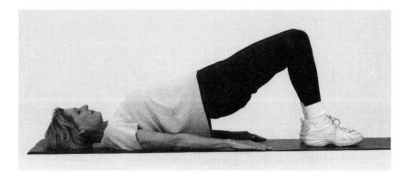

Exercise 22: Abdominals (Floor Work)

Bending in Half

PURPOSE
To strengthen the abdominals and provide core body strength. This exercise may be contraindicated for those who have had a TRAM flap. The exercise will help improve posture, which can be adversely affected by mastectomy and reconstructive surgery.

MAIN MUSCLES WORKED
Abdominals (rectus abdominis, transverse abdominis, obliques).

STARTING POSITION B

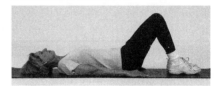

- Lie on your back
- Knees bent
- Feet flat on floor, hip width apart
- Abdominals contracted
- Small of your back pressed into the floor
- Arms straight at your sides, palms down

DESCRIPTION OF EXERCISE/PELVIC TILT
1. Flatten your lower back into the floor by contracting your abdominals and buttocks at the same time. If you have trouble with the motion, think of pressing the small of your back into the floor as if you were trying to squish a grape between your lower back and the floor. **2.** Hold the position for 5 seconds and then return to the starting position. **3.** Repeat 8–12 times.

This exercise can also be done with your legs straight or while standing (place your back against a wall if you need support while doing this exercise in a standing position).

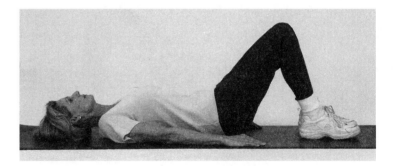

DESCRIPTION OF EXERCISE/BASIC CRUNCH

1. Tilt your pelvis so that your lower back is flat on the floor. Keeping your arms extended at your sides, slowly lift your shoulders and head off the floor using your abdominals (think of pulling your navel toward the floor). Keep your chin in a steady position (as if you were holding someone's fist in place under your chin—do not let your head fall back or tuck your chin to your chest). Do not come up so far that your lower back comes off the floor. **2.** Pause briefly. **3.** Lower yourself slowly. **4.** Repeat 8–12 times.

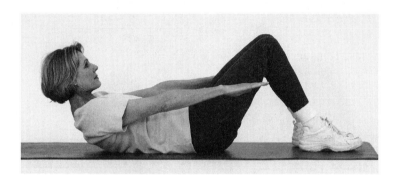

DESCRIPTION OF EXERCISE/OBLIQUE WORK

1. Perform the same exercise as the Basic Crunch but add a slight twist. As you keep your arms extended and lift your shoulders and head off the floor, reach with both hands to the outside of your right leg. **2.** Pause. **3.** Lower yourself slowly back to the floor. **4.** Perform the lift 8–12 times. **5.** Repeat the lift, reaching to the outside of the left leg.

Remember to breathe consistently throughout the exercises. Do not hold your breath. You may find it helpful to exhale as you raise yourself up and inhale as you lower yourself back down. You want to make sure that you pull your navel toward your spine as you perform the exercise. Don't let your stomach "puff out."

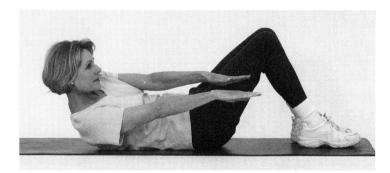

Exercise 23: Abdominals (Standing)

Cheerleader

PURPOSE
To strengthen the abdominals and provide core body strength. This exercise may not be appropriate for those who have had a TRAM flap. The exercise will help improve posture, which can be adversely affected by mastectomy and reconstructive surgery.

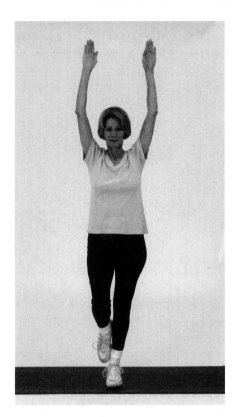

MAIN MUSCLES WORKED
Abdominals (rectus abdominis, transverse abdominis, obliques).

STARTING POSITION A

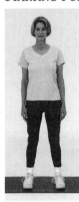

- Stand up straight
- Arms at your sides
- Feet shoulder width apart
- Knees slightly bent
- Abdominals contracted
- Lower back muscles contracted
- Shoulders down and back
- Chest lifted
- Look straight ahead

DESCRIPTION OF EXERCISE
1. Stand on one leg and hold the other leg so that your toes are resting next to the ankle of the standing leg. Contract your abdominals and buttocks to stabilize your torso. **2.** Slowly flap your arms out to the sides and up over your head like a bird in flight 8–12 times. **3.** Bring your arms to your sides, with your palms against the sides of your legs. **4.** Move your arms up and down in front of you in a scissorslike motion 8–12 times. **5.** Hold your arms

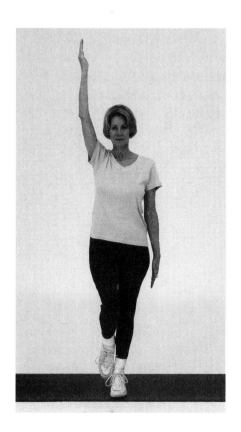
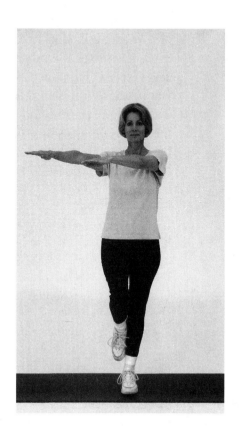

straight out in front of you at shoulder height, with your palms facing the floor. **6.** Keeping your elbows straight, move your arms together from side to side in front of you, without letting your shoulders or torso move (the only motion is at the shoulder joint), 8–12 times. **7.** Repeat steps 2–6 while standing on your other leg.

Keep breathing regularly throughout the exercise. Move your arms in a controlled manner in all steps of this exercise.

Level IV

Level IV introduces additional combination exercises in which you perform both an upper and a lower body exercise at the same time. The principles of progression are similar to those in the previous levels: begin with one set of 8–12 repetitions and progress to two to three sets of 8–12 repetitions. In some cases, you will aim for 12–15 repetitions. You also will increase the resistance you use. As with the other levels, progress slowly and at your own pace.

If you experience any pain, loss of range of motion, change in skin texture, or swelling, stop exercising and call your doctor immediately. If given the OK to continue, reduce the number of repetitions and the resistance you are using, or go back to the previous level.

Level IV Exercises

	TECHNICAL NAME	ANALOGY NAME
Exercise 1	Half-Rep Chest Fly on Floor with Weights	Hugging a Barrel
Exercise 2	Hamstring Curls with Chair	Frog Kicks
Exercise 3	Modified to Full Floor Push-ups	G.I. Jane
Exercise 4	Exercise Ball Squat with Weights	Orangutan
Exercise 5	Double-Arm Bent-Over Row with Forearm Twist	Pulling Weeds
Exercise 6	Lunge	Stepping Backward
Exercise 7	Reverse Fly	Bird Flapping Its Wings
Exercise 8	"Lat" Pull Down/Leg Lift Combo with Band	Aerobic Dancing
Exercise 9	Exercise Ball Squat/Shoulder Press Combo	Touchdown
Exercise 10	Lunge with Weights	Ballet Skiing
Exercise 11	Exercise Ball Squat with Frontal Raise	Riding a Motorcycle
Exercise 12	Isometric Adductors with Upright Row	Zipping Up My Zipper
Exercise 13	Lunge/Arm Curl Combo with Weights	Superhero Lifting a Car
Exercise 14	Plié/Overhead Extension Combo with Weight	Pouring Water Down Your Back

Exercise 15	Biceps Curl/Triceps Kick Back Combo with Weights	Indecision
Exercise 16	Traffic Cop	Traffic Cop
Exercise 17	Serratus Reach with Weight	Reaching for the Stars
Exercise 18	Lower Back (Floor Work)	Modified Superwoman
Exercise 19	Lower Back (Floor Work)	Superwoman
Exercise 20	Lower Back (Floor Work)	Bridging
Exercise 21	Bridging with Variations	Building My Bridge to the Future
Exercise 22	Abdominals (Floor Work)	Bending in Half
Exercise 23	Abdominals (Standing)	Cheerleader

Level
IV

Exercise 1: Half-Rep Chest Fly on Floor with Weights

Hugging a Barrel

PURPOSE
To stretch your incision and skin across the chest wall and to strengthen the chest muscles.

MAIN MUSCLES WORKED
Chest (pectorals), shoulders (anterior deltoids), back of upper arms (triceps), and a shoulder girdle muscle (serratus anterior).

STARTING POSITION B

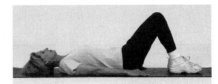

- Lie on your back
- Knees bent
- Feet flat on floor, hip width apart
- Abdominals contracted
- Small of your back pressed into the floor
- Arms straight at your sides, palms down

DESCRIPTION OF EXERCISE
1. Hold a 1- to 5-pound weight in each hand. Raise your hands straight up in the air above your chest, with your palms facing each other. Hold your shoulder blades down and back against the floor (see top photo on page 121). **2.** Keeping a slight bend in your elbows, slowly lower your arms out to the sides as far as is comfortable (pretend you are holding a barrel in your arms). **3.** Raise your arms 2 inches, then lower them back down. **4.** Contract your chest, feeling the tension in your armpits, then bring your arms back up above your chest. **5.** Repeat steps 2–4, 8–12 times.

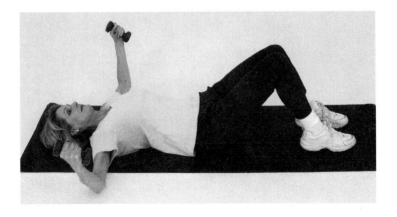

Exercise 2: Hamstring Curls with Chair

Frog Kicks

PURPOSE

To increase lower body strength used in everyday activities such as sitting, standing, and walking and to maintain functional independence.

MAIN MUSCLES WORKED

Back of thighs (hamstrings), buttocks (gluteals), abdominals, and lower back (erector spinae).

STARTING POSITION B

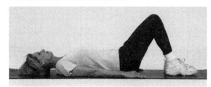

• Lie on your back
• Knees bent
• Feet flat on floor, hip width apart
• Abdominals contracted
• Small of your back pressed into the floor
• Arms straight at your sides, palms down

DESCRIPTION OF EXERCISE

1. Bend your knees at a 90-degree angle and place your heels shoulder width apart on a chair. **2.** Exhale as you push your heels into the chair and raise your hips up off the floor. **3.** Inhale as you return to the starting position. **4.** Repeat 8–12 times.

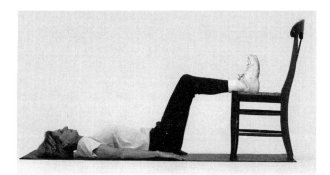

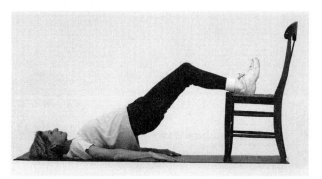

Exercise 3: Modified to Full Floor Push-ups

G.I. Jane

PURPOSE
To strengthen the muscles of the chest wall and improve upper body range of motion.

MAIN MUSCLES WORKED
Chest (pectorals), front of shoulders (anterior deltoids), back of upper arms (triceps), and a shoulder girdle muscle (serratus anterior).

STARTING POSITION C

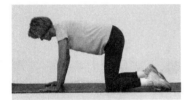

- On hands and knees
- Hands directly beneath shoulders (fingers face forward)
- Arms straight but not locked
- Knees shoulder width apart
- Head and neck a natural extension of the spine

DESCRIPTION OF EXERCISE
1. Get on the floor on your hands and knees. Walk your hands forward so that your back is flat. (Your body should form a straight line from your head to your knees.) Keep your head aligned with your spine, your abdominals contracted, and your back flat throughout the exercise. **2.** Inhale as you lower yourself toward the floor, to within 3–5 inches of the floor (or as far as is comfortable), by bending your elbows. Be sure to contract your abdominals and squeeze your buttocks to stabilize your torso. Don't let your back droop. If you feel pain in your lower back, adjust your position. **3.** Contract your chest muscles (imagine squeezing a banana under each armpit) and push yourself away from the floor by straightening your elbows (be sure not to lock them). **4.** Repeat 8–12 times.

For an extra challenge, straighten your legs completely and get up on your toes in step 1. If you have any pain with this exercise, do not do it. Instead, return to a chest exercise from a previous level. If you have had an axillary node dissection, monitor your arm's response to these push-ups to ensure that you do not overdo it.

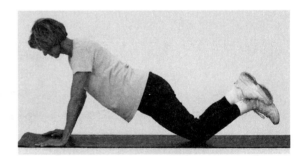

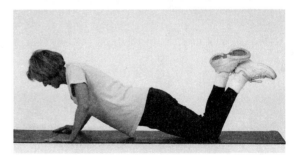

Exercise 4: Exercise Ball Squat with Weights

Orangutan

PURPOSE
To improve posture and balance, strengthen and stabilize the torso, and strengthen the lower body. You will use your abdominals and buttocks (gluteals) during this exercise to stabilize your torso, which will help protect your lower back from injury. You will also use muscles involved in pelvic stabilization and everyday activities such as sitting, standing, and walking.

MAIN MUSCLES WORKED
Front of thighs (quadriceps), back of thighs (hamstrings), and buttocks (gluteals).

STARTING POSITION A

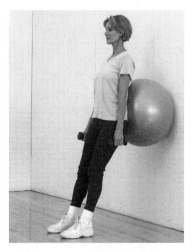

- Stand up straight
- Arms at your sides
- Feet shoulder width apart
- Knees slightly bent
- Abdominals contracted
- Lower back muscles contracted
- Shoulders down and back
- Chest lifted
- Look straight ahead

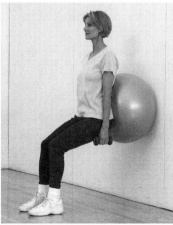

DESCRIPTION OF EXERCISE
1. Stand near the wall with an exercise ball in the small of your back and against the wall. Walk your legs out about 18 inches, keeping your feet shoulder width apart and your toes pointing forward. Hold a 1- to 5-pound weight in each hand and let your arms hang by your sides, with your palms facing your thighs. Do not lock your elbows. **2.** Inhale as you press back firmly against the ball and lower your torso by bending your knees. Go as low as you comfortably can, but no lower than with your knees bent at a 90-degree angle. Do not let your knees go past your toes. (Try to keep your knees over your ankles.) **3.** Exhale as you straighten your legs and return to the starting position. Do not lock your knees. Keep your head and neck straight and look forward. **4.** Repeat 8–12 times.

If it feels more natural for you, breathe in the opposite pattern from that described above.

Level
IV

Pulling Weeds

PURPOSE
To strengthen the back and improve range
of motion.

MAIN MUSCLES WORKED
Upper back (rhomboids), back of shoulders (posterior deltoids), and front of
upper arms (biceps).

STARTING POSITION
See "Description of Exercise."

DESCRIPTION OF EXERCISE
1. Sit forward on a chair or bench with
your knees bent at a 90-degree angle and
your feet together, flat on the floor. Hold a
1- to 5-pound weight in each hand. **2.** Lean
forward from your hips and support your
torso on your thighs. Keep your head and
neck aligned with your spine. Let your
arms hang down from your shoulders,
with your palms facing behind you and
your hands near your feet. **3.** Bend your
elbows as you raise your arms up and
back, squeezing your shoulder blades and
lifting the weights to hip level. Keep your
elbows close to your sides. **4.** Keeping your
shoulder blades together, rotate your
hands so that your palms face forward
(up). **5.** Lower your arms to the starting
position, rotating your hands so that your
palms face backward again. Feel the
stretch across your upper back. **6.** Repeat
8–12 times.

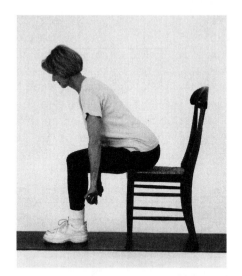

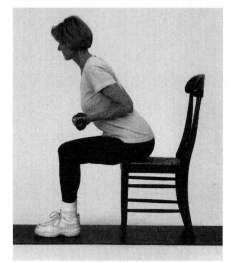

Exercise 6: Lunge

Stepping Backward

PURPOSE
To strengthen the muscles of the lower body while providing balance and stability training.

MAIN MUSCLES WORKED
Front of thighs (quadriceps), back of thighs (hamstrings), buttocks (gluteals), abdominals, and lower back (erector spinae).

STARTING POSITION A

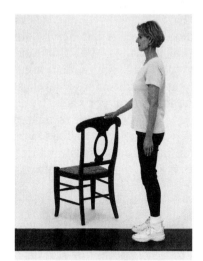

- Stand up straight
- Arms at your sides
- Feet shoulder width apart
- Knees slightly bent
- Abdominals contracted
- Lower back muscles contracted
- Shoulders down and back
- Chest lifted
- Look straight ahead

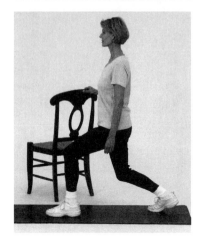

DESCRIPTION OF EXERCISE
1. Stand next to a chair. Take a step backward with your right foot so that it is 2–3 feet in back of the left and your feet are hip width apart. Your hips should be directly under your shoulders and your torso upright. Your arms hang by your sides or rest on your hips. **2.** Bend both knees so that your left knee is over your left ankle, your left lower leg is perpendicular to the floor, your right lower leg is parallel to the floor, and your right heel is lifted. Both legs should be bent at 90 degrees. (If they are not, adjust the position of your feet.) Keep your abdominals contracted, your rib cage lifted, and your torso upright. **3.** Squeeze your buttocks and straighten both legs to raise yourself back up to the step 1 position. **4.** Repeat 8–12 times. **5.** Repeat steps 1–4 with your right foot forward. Keep breathing!

If 90 degrees is too difficult for you, start by lowering yourself a quarter of the way down.

Level IV

Exercise 7: Reverse Fly

Bird Flapping Its Wings

PURPOSE
To promote muscular balance by strengthening the back of the shoulders and improve posture and reduce hunchback by increasing muscular awareness and strengthening the upper back. Hunchback can occur after surgery due to tightening in the chest wall. Seek the advice of your doctor if you have had a latissimus dorsi flap or if you have lower back problems.

MAIN MUSCLES WORKED
Back (rhomboids, middle trapezius, latissimus dorsi) and shoulders (posterior and medial deltoids).

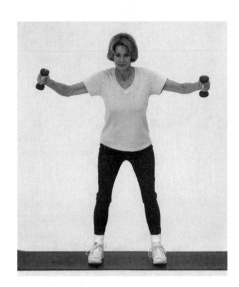

STARTING POSITION A

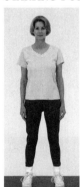

- Stand up straight
- Arms at your sides
- Feet shoulder width apart
- Knees slightly bent
- Abdominals contracted
- Lower back muscles contracted
- Shoulders down and back
- Chest lifted
- Look straight ahead

DESCRIPTION OF EXERCISE
1. Hold a 1- to 5-pound weight in each hand. **2.** Contract your abdominals and, keeping your back flat and your head aligned with your spine, bend over from the hips at a 30- to 45-degree angle. Let your arms hang straight down from your shoulders, with your palms facing in and your elbows slightly bent. Pull your shoulder blades down and back and hold them there. If the standing position is too stressful on your back, sit on the edge of a chair and bend forward from your hips, keeping your back straight and your head and neck aligned. Support your torso on your thighs and let your arms hang down from your shoulders with your palms facing in. Continue the exercise as in the standing position. **3.** Exhale as you raise your arms out to the sides and up to shoulder height, maintaining your starting position with your torso. Lead with your elbows (which remain slightly bent) as your arms follow an arclike pattern. Keep your palms facing down and keep your wrists straight. **4.** Pause. **5.** Keeping the shoulder blades anchored, inhale as you slowly lower your arms back to the starting position. **6.** Repeat 8–12 times.

This exercise can also be done with an exercise band. Stand on the band and hold the handles in your hands.

Exercise 8: "Lat" Pull Down/Leg Lift Combo with Band

Level
IV

Aerobic Dancing

PURPOSE

To improve posture by increasing muscular awareness and strengthening of the upper back, reduce hunchback (kyphosis), and strengthen the large latissimus dorsi muscle, which is used in pulling motions. Be cautious if you have had a latissimus dorsi flap. The exercise also includes leg strengthening and balance work.

MAIN MUSCLES WORKED

Upper and middle back (latissimus dorsi, teres major, middle/lower trapezius, rhomboids), back of shoulders (posterior deltoids), front of upper arms (biceps), and hip flexors.

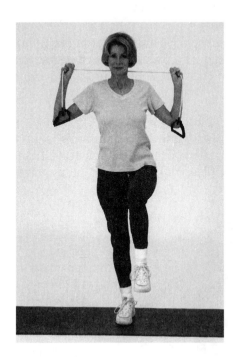

STARTING POSITION A

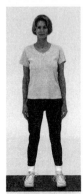

- Stand up straight
- Arms at your sides
- Feet shoulder width apart
- Knees slightly bent
- Abdominals contracted
- Lower back muscles contracted
- Shoulders down and back
- Chest lifted
- Look straight ahead

DESCRIPTION OF EXERCISE

1. Hold an exercise band stretched taut between your hands and raise your arms overhead. Your palms should face forward, and your hands should be a little wider than shoulder width apart. **2.** Pulling your shoulder blades down and together, exhale as you bend your elbows, pull the band down behind your head, and lift one knee toward your chest. Your hands should stay slightly wider than shoulder width apart and your head stays still. You will be standing on one leg. Keep your abdominals contracted and your chest lifted. **3.** Inhale as you lower your leg and raise your arms back to the starting position. **4.** Repeat, lifting the other leg as you pull your arms down. **5.** Repeat steps 2–4, 8–12 times.

If you use a weight machine to perform this exercise, pull the bar in front of you, not behind your head. Keep your head and neck straight and aligned with your spine.

Exercise 9: Exercise Ball Squat/Shoulder Press Combo

Touchdown

PURPOSE
To improve posture by promoting muscle strength and awareness, reduce swayback, strengthen the lower back, and improve stabilization of the body core.

MAIN MUSCLES WORKED
Buttocks (gluteals), front of thighs (quadriceps), back of thighs (hamstrings), shoulders (deltoids), and back of upper arms (triceps brachii).

STARTING POSITION A

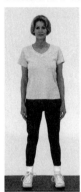

- Stand up straight
- Arms at your sides
- Feet shoulder width apart
- Knees slightly bent
- Abdominals contracted
- Lower back muscles contracted
- Shoulders down and back
- Chest lifted
- Look straight ahead

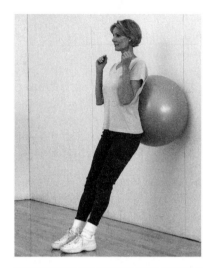

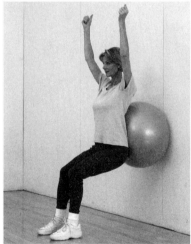

DESCRIPTION OF EXERCISE
1. Stand near the wall with an exercise ball in the small of your back and against the wall. Walk your legs out about 18 inches, keeping your feet shoulder width apart and your toes pointing forward. Bend your elbows so that your hands are up near your shoulders with your palms facing each other. **2.** Inhale as you press back firmly against the ball and lower your body by bending your knees. Go as low as you comfortably can, but no lower than with your knees bent at a 90-degree angle. Keep your knees over your ankles. As you lower yourself, raise your arms up overhead.

3. Exhale as you straighten your legs and lower your arms back to the starting position. Do not lock your knees or elbows. Keep your head and neck straight and look forward. **4.** Repeat 8–12 times.

If it feels more natural for you, breathe in the opposite pattern from that described above.

Exercise 10: Lunge with Weights

Ballet Skiing

PURPOSE
To improve posture and balance, strengthen and stabilize the torso, and improve lower body strength and range of motion. Stabilizing your torso will help protect your lower back from injury and strengthen the muscles used in everyday activities such as sitting, standing, and walking.

MAIN MUSCLES WORKED
Buttocks (gluteals), back of thighs (hamstrings), and front of thighs (quadriceps).

STARTING POSITION A

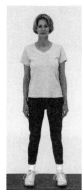

- Stand up straight
- Arms at your sides
- Feet shoulder width apart
- Knees slightly bent
- Abdominals contracted
- Lower back muscles contracted
- Shoulders down and back
- Chest lifted
- Look straight ahead

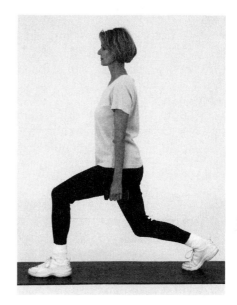

DESCRIPTION OF EXERCISE
1. Hold a 1- to 5-pound weight in each hand. **2.** Take a step forward with your left foot so that it is 2–3 feet in front of the right and your feet are hip width apart. Your hips should be directly under your shoulders and your torso upright. Your arms hang by your sides, with your elbows slightly bent and your palms facing in. **3.** Bend both knees so that your left knee is over your left ankle, your left lower leg is perpendicular to the floor, your right lower leg is parallel to the floor, and your right heel is lifted. Both legs should be bent at 90 degrees. (If they are not, adjust the position of your feet.) Keep your abdominals contracted, your rib cage lifted, and your torso upright. **4.** Squeeze your buttocks and straighten both legs to raise yourself back up to the step 2 position. **5.** Repeat 8–12 times. **6.** Repeat steps 2–5 with your right foot forward. Keep breathing!

If 90 degrees is too difficult for you, start by lowering yourself a quarter of the way down.

Level
IV

Exercise 11: Exercise Ball Squat with Frontal Arm Raise

Riding a Motorcycle

PURPOSE
To improve lower body strength, increase range of motion in the shoulder, and improve shoulder strength and stability.

MAIN MUSCLES WORKED
Buttocks (gluteals), front of thighs (quadriceps), back of thighs (hamstrings), and front of shoulders (anterior deltoids).

STARTING POSITION
See "Description of Exercise."

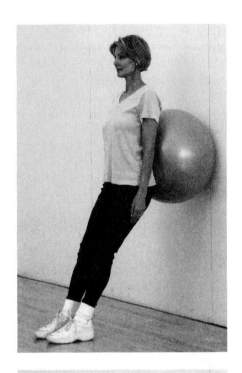

DESCRIPTION OF EXERCISE
1. Stand near the wall with an exercise ball in the small of your back and against the wall. Walk your legs out about 18 inches, keeping your feet shoulder width apart and your toes pointing forward. Your arms should hang by your sides, with your palms facing your thighs. **2.** Inhale as you press back firmly against the ball and lower your body by bending your knees. Go as low as you comfortably can, but no lower than with your knees bent at a 90-degree angle. Make sure your knees do not go past your toes. (Try to keep your knees over your ankles.) As you lower yourself, raise your arms out in front of you to shoulder height. **3.** Exhale as you straighten your legs, squeeze your buttocks, and lower your arms back to the starting position. Do not lock your knees or elbows. Keep your head and neck straight and look forward. **4.** Repeat 8–12 times.

If it feels more natural for you, breathe in the opposite pattern from that described above.

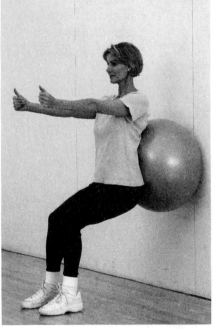

Exercise 12: Isometric Adductors with Upright Row

Level

IV

Zipping Up My Zipper

PURPOSE
To strengthen the muscles of the inner thighs and to strengthen the muscles of the upper back to help improve posture and stabilize the shoulder girdle.

MAIN MUSCLES WORKED
Inside of thighs (adductors), upper back (upper trapezius), and shoulders (deltoids).

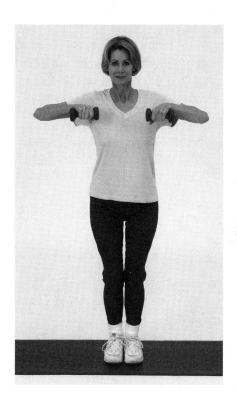

STARTING POSITION F

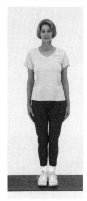

- Stand up straight
- Arms at your sides
- Feet together
- Knees slightly bent
- Abdominals contracted
- Lower back muscles contracted
- Shoulders down and back
- Chest lifted
- Look straight ahead

DESCRIPTION OF EXERCISE
1. Hold a 1- to 5-pound weight in each hand. Let your arms hang in front of your body, with your palms facing your thighs and the weights about 6 inches apart. **2.** Squeeze your legs together as tight as you can as you exhale and bend your elbows to bring your hands up toward your chin. Keep your hands close to your body; your wrists will turn slightly. At the end of the movement, your elbows should be at shoulder height, not above. Keep your back straight and do not rock or sway during the movement. Do not hold your breath. **3.** Continue squeezing your legs together and inhale as you lower your hands back to the starting position. Do not lock your elbows. **4.** Repeat 8–12 times, relaxing your legs between repetitions.

This exercise can also be done with an exercise band. Place the band under your feet and hold the handles in your hands.

Level
IV

Exercise 13: Lunge/Arm Curl Combo with Weights

Superhero Lifting a Car

PURPOSE
To improve balance, improve torso stability, and strengthen muscles involved in everyday activities such as sitting, standing, walking, pulling, and carrying.

MAIN MUSCLES WORKED
Front of thighs (quadriceps), back of thighs (hamstrings), buttocks (gluteals), and front of upper arms (biceps).

STARTING POSITION A

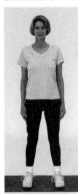

- Stand up straight
- Arms at your sides
- Feet shoulder width apart
- Knees slightly bent
- Abdominals contracted
- Lower back muscles contracted
- Shoulders down and back
- Chest lifted
- Look straight ahead

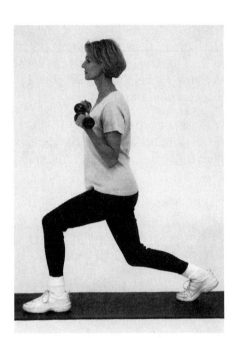

DESCRIPTION OF EXERCISE
1. Hold a 1- to 5-pound weight in each hand. **2.** Take a step forward with your left foot so that it is 2–3 feet in front of the right and your feet are hip width apart. Your hips should be directly under your shoulders and your torso upright. Your arms hang by your sides, with your palms facing forward. Pull your shoulder blades down and back. **3.** Exhale as you bend both knees to a 90-degree angle, lowering yourself toward the floor. Bend both elbows, curling your forearms toward your upper arms. Your left knee is over your left ankle, your right lower leg is parallel to the floor, your right heel is lifted, and your elbows stay directly under your shoulders. Keep your weight on the heel in front and the toes in back. Keep your abdominals contracted, your rib cage lifted, your head up, and your torso over your hips. Do not lean forward as you lower yourself. Keep your wrists rigid and press your elbows and upper arms into your body as you lift your forearms. **4.** Inhale as you straighten your knees and lower your arms to the starting position. **5.** Repeat 8–12 times, staying in the lunge position throughout. **6.** Repeat steps 2–5 with the right leg.

This exercise can also be done with an exercise band. Place the band under your front foot and hold the handles in your hands.

Exercise 14: Plié/Overhead Extension Combo with Weight
Level IV

Pouring Water Down Your Back

PURPOSE
To improve balance, strengthen the torso, and strengthen muscles used in everyday activities such as sitting, standing, walking, and brushing your hair.

MAIN MUSCLES WORKED
Front of thighs (quadriceps), back of thighs (hamstrings), buttocks (gluteals), some inner thighs (adductors), and back of upper arms (triceps).

STARTING POSITION E

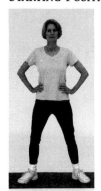

- Stand up straight
- Hands on hips
- Feet wider than shoulder width apart
- Toes turned out slightly to the side
- Knees slightly bent
- Abdominals contracted
- Lower back muscles contracted
- Shoulders down and back
- Chest lifted
- Look straight ahead

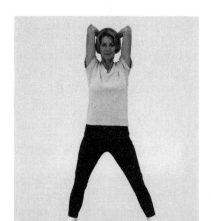

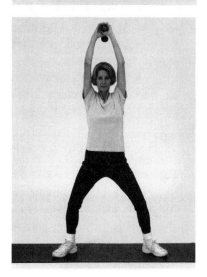

DESCRIPTION OF EXERCISE
1. Hold a 1- to 5-pound weight with both hands (the weight should hang down vertically). Raise your arms up over your head and bend your elbows so that your hands are behind your head and your elbows point directly up toward the ceiling. Keep your elbows close to your head. **2.** Exhale as you bend your knees and lower your torso (buttocks) down as far as you can go, but no lower than with your thighs parallel to the floor. Make sure your knees don't go past your toes. As you bend your knees, straighten your arms so that your hands are above your head. Keep your upper arms beside your ears. Keep your abdomen contracted and your back straight. Do not bend forward or backward. **3.** Inhale as you return to the starting position by straightening your knees and bending your elbows. **4.** Repeat 8–12 times.

Level IV

Exercise 15: Biceps Curl/Triceps Kick Back Combo with Weights

Indecision

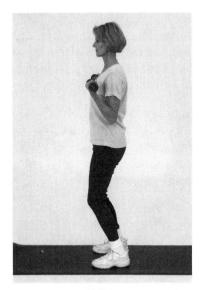

PURPOSE
To increase upper arm strength for performing everyday activities involving pushing and pulling motions (pushing up off of a chair, brushing your hair, opening a door).

MAIN MUSCLES WORKED
Front of upper arms (biceps) and back of upper arms (triceps).

STARTING POSITION A

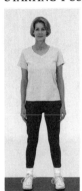

- Stand up straight
- Arms at your sides
- Feet shoulder width apart
- Knees slightly bent
- Abdominals contracted
- Lower back muscles contracted
- Shoulders down and back
- Chest lifted
- Look straight ahead

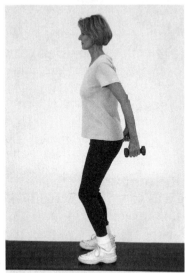

DESCRIPTION OF EXERCISE
1. Hold a 1- to 5-pound weight in each hand, with your arms hanging at your sides and your palms facing forward. **2.** Holding your elbows close to your sides and under your shoulders, exhale and curl both arms toward your shoulders. **3.** Inhale as you lower your arms to the starting position. **4.** Turn your hands so that your palms face in. **5.** Exhale as you push your arms back behind you, keeping your elbows close by your sides. As you push your arms back, your palms should continue to face each other. **6.** Inhale as you return to the starting position. **7.** Repeat steps 2–6, 8–12 times.

Do not sway, bend, or lean in any direction as you perform the exercise. Keep your shoulders down and back and your neck relaxed throughout the exercise.

Exercise 16: Traffic Cop   Level

Traffic Cop

PURPOSE
To increase range of motion in external shoulder rotation, strengthen the rotator cuff, and improve stability of the shoulder joint.

MAIN MUSCLES WORKED
Back of shoulders (posterior deltoids) and some rotator cuff muscles (infraspinatus, teres minor).

STARTING POSITION A

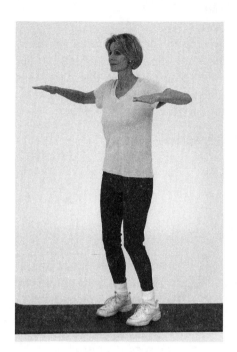

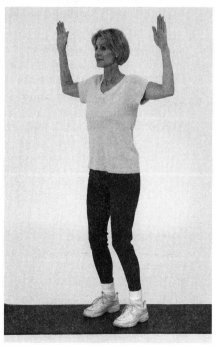

* Stand up straight
* Arms at your sides
* Feet shoulder width apart
* Knees slightly bent
* Abdominals contracted
* Lower back muscles contracted
* Shoulders down and back
* Chest lifted
* Look straight ahead

DESCRIPTION OF EXERCISE
1. Bend your elbows 90 degrees and raise your arms out to the sides at shoulder height, so that your forearms and upper arms are parallel to the floor. (Your palms should be facing the floor.) **2.** Keeping your upper arms parallel to the floor, exhale as you rotate your arms upward until your forearms are perpendicular to the floor. (Your palms will be facing forward.) **3.** Inhale as you slowly lower your arms to the starting position. Keep your back straight, your abdominals tight, and your shoulder blades down and back. Do not rock or sway. **4.** Perform 8–12 repetitions.

Do not use weights with this exercise.

Exercise 17: Serratus Reach with Weight

Reaching for the Stars

PURPOSE

To strengthen the serratus anterior muscle of the shoulder girdle, which holds the shoulder blade against the back, and to prevent feelings of weakness in the arm when reaching in front of you.

MAIN MUSCLES WORKED

A shoulder girdle muscle (serratus anterior).

STARTING POSITION B

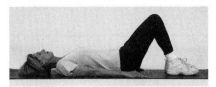

- Lie on your back
- Knees bent
- Feet flat on floor, hip width apart
- Abdominals contracted
- Small of your back pressed into the floor
- Arms straight at your sides, palms down

DESCRIPTION OF EXERCISE

1. Hold a 1- to 5-pound weight in your hands. Raise your arms so that they are pointing straight up toward the ceiling (perpendicular to the floor), with your palms facing in. (If you are holding a weight in each hand, your palms face your feet.) **2.** Exhale and inhale as you reach for the ceiling in three steps by raising your arms up slightly and holding that position, then raising them slightly higher and holding that position, and finally raising them as high as you can, lifting your shoulders off the floor. Keep your elbows straight and your head aligned with your spine, looking up at the ceiling. **3.** Hold your arms up for 5 seconds. **4.** Inhale as you lower your arms back to the starting position. **5.** Repeat steps 2–4, 8–12 times.

Your head and back stay on the floor throughout the exercise; only your shoulders lift up as you reach for the ceiling. Remember to breathe continuously throughout the exercise.

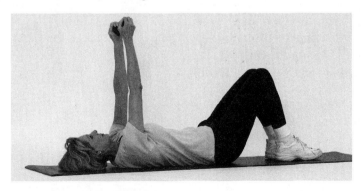

Exercise 18: Lower Back (Floor Work)   Level
                                                            IV

Modified Superwoman

PURPOSE

To strengthen the lower back and develop core body strength. This exercise is particularly beneficial for those who have had a TRAM flap. With any of the back exercises, stop if you feel any pain.

MAIN MUSCLES WORKED

Lower back (erector spinae), back of thighs (hamstrings), and buttocks (gluteals).

STARTING POSITION C

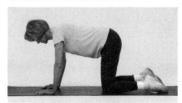

- On hands and knees
- Hands directly beneath shoulders (fingers face forward)
- Arms straight but not locked
- Knees shoulder width apart
- Head and neck a natural extension of the spine

DESCRIPTION OF EXERCISE

1. Raise your right arm straight out in front of you, no higher than shoulder level, and your left leg straight out behind you, no higher than hip level. Your body should be parallel to the floor. Squeeze your buttocks and contract your abdominals. Keep your head aligned with your spine, looking straight down. **2.** Hold the position for 5 seconds. **3.** Relax your buttocks and abdominals as you lower your arm and leg. **4.** Repeat the entire exercise with your left arm and right leg. **5.** Repeat steps 1–4, 6 times.

Remember to breathe consistently throughout the exercise. Do not hold your breath.

If you have any pain on your affected side, do not do this exercise but move on to Exercise 19.

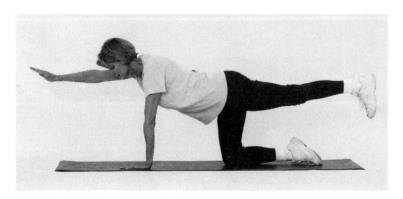

Exercise 19: Lower Back (Floor Work)

Superwoman

PURPOSE
To strengthen the lower back and develop core body strength. This exercise is particularly beneficial for those who have had a TRAM flap. With any of the back exercises, stop if you feel any pain.

MAIN MUSCLES WORKED
Lower back (erector spinae), back of thighs (hamstrings), and buttocks (gluteals).

STARTING POSITION
See "Description of Exercise."

DESCRIPTION OF EXERCISE
1. Lie facedown on the floor with your arms straight out in front of you. You may place a pillow or rolled-up towel under your forehead to keep your head and neck aligned with your spine. 2. Contract your abdominals and squeeze your buttocks. 3. Raise your right arm and left leg off the floor. Your head and chest will come up off the floor, but you will continue to look down, keeping your head and neck aligned with your spine. 4. Hold for 5 seconds. 5. Lower your arm and leg. 6. Repeat with your left arm and right leg. 7. Repeat steps 2–6, 8–12 times.

If needed, you can place a pillow under your chest and stomach or raise yourself up on one arm.

Remember to breathe consistently throughout the exercise. Do not hold your breath.

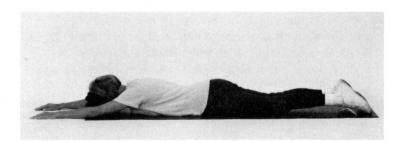

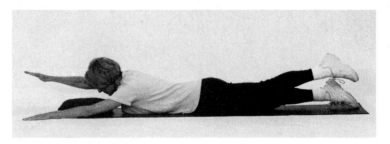

Exercise 20: Lower Back (Floor Work)

Bridging

PURPOSE

To strengthen the lower back and develop core body strength. This exercise is particularly beneficial for those who have had a TRAM flap. With any of the back exercises, stop if you feel any pain.

MAIN MUSCLES WORKED

Lower back (erector spinae), back of thighs (hamstrings), and buttocks (gluteals).

STARTING POSITION B

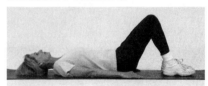

- Lie on your back
- Knees bent
- Feet flat on floor, hip width apart
- Abdominals contracted
- Small of your back pressed into the floor
- Arms straight at your sides, palms down

DESCRIPTION OF EXERCISE

1. Raise your hips (pelvis) off the floor by contracting your abdominals, lower back, and buttocks until your body forms a straight line from your kneecaps and thighs to your chin. Be sure to keep your shoulders and upper back in contact with the floor. **2.** Keeping your pelvis level, hold the straight-line position for 5 seconds. **3.** Lower your hips to about 3 inches above the floor. **4.** Repeat 8–12 times.

Remember to breathe consistently throughout the exercise. Do not hold your breath.

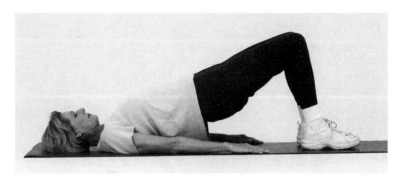

Level
IV

Exercise 21: Bridging with Variations

Building My Bridge to the Future

PURPOSE

To strengthen the lower back and develop core body strength. This exercise is particularly beneficial for those who have had a TRAM flap. Additionally, it can help improve posture, which can be adversely affected by mastectomy and reconstructive surgery. With any of the back exercises, stop if you feel any pain.

MAIN MUSCLES WORKED

Lower back (erector spinae), buttocks (gluteals), back of thighs (hamstrings), front of thighs (quadriceps), and abdominals.

STARTING POSITION B

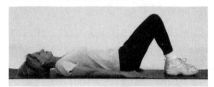

- Lie on your back
- Knees bent
- Feet flat on floor, hip width apart
- Abdominals contracted
- Small of your back pressed into the floor
- Arms straight at your sides, palms down

DESCRIPTION OF EXERCISE/BRIDGING WITH LEG EXTENSION

1. Raise your hips (pelvis) off the floor by contracting your abdominals, lower back, and buttocks until your body forms a straight line from your kneecaps and thighs to your chin. Be sure to keep your shoulders and upper back in contact with the floor. **2.** Keeping your pelvis level, lift one foot off the floor and straighten the leg. **3.** Pause for 1 or 2 seconds. **4.** Inhale as you lower your leg and straighten the other leg. **5.** Pause for 1 or 2 seconds. **6.** Lower your hips back to the floor. **7.** Repeat 8–12 times.

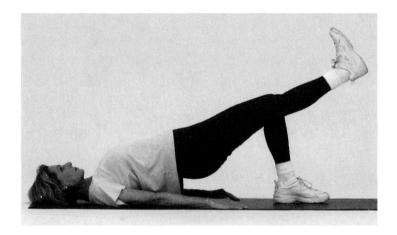

DESCRIPTION OF EXERCISE/BRIDGING WITH ADDUCTOR SQUEEZE

Level IV

1. Move your feet and legs together, keeping your feet flat on the floor. **2.** Exhale as you raise your hips (pelvis) off the floor by contracting your buttocks and squeezing your legs together until your body forms a straight line from your kneecaps and thighs to your chin. Be sure to keep your shoulders and upper back in contact with the floor. **3.** Inhale as you relax your buttocks and legs and lower your hips to about 3 inches above the floor. **4.** Repeat steps 2 and 3, 8–12 times.

Remember to breathe consistently throughout the exercises. Do not hold your breath.

You may also perform this exercise by placing a ball between your legs and squeezing it as shown in the photograph.

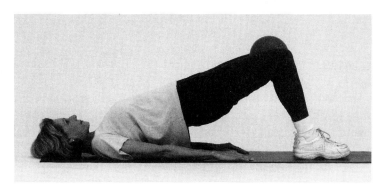

Level
IV

Exercise 22: Abdominals (Floor Work)

Bending in Half

PURPOSE
To strengthen the abdominals and provide
core body strength. This exercise may be
contraindicated for those who have had a
TRAM flap. The exercise will help improve
posture, which can be adversely affected
by mastectomy and reconstructive surgery.

MAIN MUSCLES WORKED
Abdominals (rectus abdominis, transverse
abdominis, obliques).

STARTING POSITION B

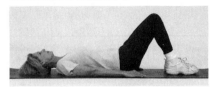

- Lie on your back
- Knees bent
- Feet flat on floor, hip width apart
- Abdominals contracted
- Small of your back pressed into the
  floor
- Arms straight at your sides, palms
  down

DESCRIPTION OF EXERCISE/PELVIC TILT
1. Flatten your lower back into the floor by contracting your abdominals and buttocks at the same time. If you have trouble with the
motion, think of pressing the small of your back into the floor as if
you were trying to squish a grape between your lower back and the
floor. **2.** Hold the position for 5 seconds and then return to the starting position. **3.** Repeat 8–12 times.

This exercise can also be done with your legs straight or while standing (place your back against a wall if you need support while doing
this exercise in a standing position).

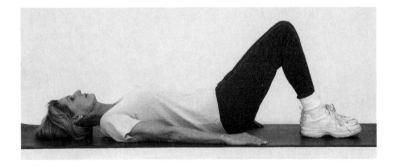

DESCRIPTION OF EXERCISE/BASIC CRUNCH

Level
IV

1. Tilt your pelvis so that your lower back is flat on the floor. Keeping your arms extended at your sides, slowly lift your shoulders and head off the floor using your abdominals (think of pulling your navel toward the floor). Keep your chin in a steady position (as if you were holding someone's fist in place under your chin—do not let your head fall back or tuck your chin to your chest). Do not come up so far that your lower back comes off the floor. **2.** Pause briefly. **3.** Lower yourself slowly. **4.** Repeat 8–12 times.

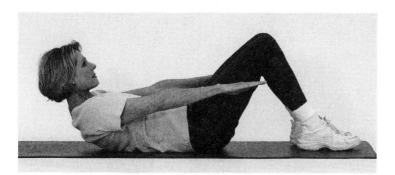

DESCRIPTION OF EXERCISE/OBLIQUE WORK

1. Perform the same exercise as the Basic Crunch but add a slight twist. As you keep your arms extended and lift your shoulders and head off the floor, reach with both hands to the outside of your right leg. **2.** Pause. **3.** Lower yourself slowly back to the floor. **4.** Perform the lift 8–12 times. **5.** Repeat the lift, reaching to the outside of the left leg.

Remember to breathe consistently throughout the exercises. Do not hold your breath. You may find it helpful to exhale as you raise yourself up and inhale as you lower yourself back down. You want to make sure that you pull your navel toward your spine as you perform the exercise. Don't let your stomach "puff out."

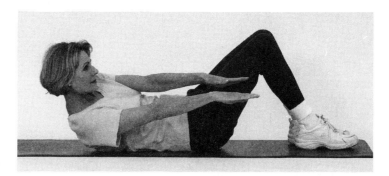

Level
IV

Exercise 23: Abdominals (Standing)

Cheerleader

PURPOSE
To strengthen the abdominals and provide core body strength. This exercise may not be appropriate for those who have had a TRAM flap. The exercise will help improve posture, which can be adversely affected by mastectomy and reconstructive surgery.

MAIN MUSCLES WORKED
Abdominals (rectus abdominis, transverse abdominis, obliques).

STARTING POSITION A

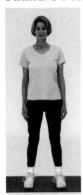

- Stand up straight
- Arms at your sides
- Feet shoulder width apart
- Knees slightly bent
- Abdominals contracted
- Lower back muscles contracted
- Shoulders down and back
- Chest lifted
- Look straight ahead

DESCRIPTION OF EXERCISE
1. Stand on one leg and hold the other leg so that your toes are resting next to the ankle of the standing leg. Contract your abdominals and buttocks to stabilize your torso. 2. Slowly flap your arms out to the sides and up over your head like a bird in flight 8–12 times. 3. Bring your arms to your sides, with your palms against the sides of your legs. 4. Move your arms up and down in front of you in a scissorslike motion 8–12 times. 5. Hold your arms

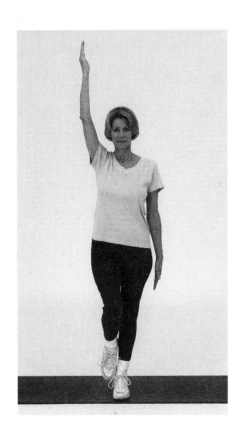
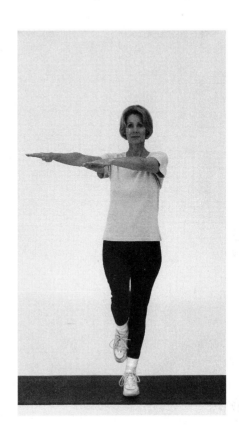

straight out in front of you at shoulder height, with your palms facing the floor. **6.** Keeping your elbows straight, move your arms together from side to side in front of you, without letting your shoulders or torso move (the only motion is at the shoulder joint), 8–12 times. **7.** Repeat steps 2–6 while standing on your other leg.

Keep breathing regularly throughout the exercise. Move your arms in a controlled manner in all steps of this exercise.

PART III

Expanding Your Exercise Program

CHAPTER 5

Am I Ready for Aerobic Exercise?

It has been proven that regular physical exercise has numerous health benefits. I consider my exercise program . . . to be just as essential in my long-term healing process from breast cancer as my chemotherapy and radiation treatments.

                              Anne Gurvin, Breast Cancer Survivor

Hope is itself a species of happiness, and, perhaps, the chief happiness which this world affords.   *—Samuel Johnson*

IN CHAPTER 1, we discussed the benefits of exercise in general. Regular exercise and a well-balanced diet can help you live a healthier, more productive life. Exercise makes you stronger, helps you manage your weight, and reduces your risk of developing many diseases. It can also make you feel less depressed and more self-confident.

The *Essential Exercises* program in Chapter 4 addresses your particular needs, as a breast cancer survivor, for flexibility and strength. This chapter helps you add aerobic exercise to your regimen, enhancing your cardiovascular function so that you will enjoy even greater benefits from exercising.

All types of fitness training—aerobic, strength, and flexibility—are based on the overload principle. This means that to strengthen one of the body's systems (muscular, cardiovascular, or respiratory), you must make that sys-

174

tem work harder than it is used to working. This process of stress and adaptation improves your physical fitness level. We feel that the same idea applies to the mind as to the body and that you, as a breast cancer survivor, have one of the strongest emotional systems around. It has certainly been put to the "overload test" through your breast cancer experience, and you are much stronger as a result.

What Aerobic Means

Aerobic, or cardiovascular, endurance describes the body's ability to take in, transport, and use oxygen, a process involving the heart and blood vessels (cardiovascular system), the lungs (respiratory system), and the muscles (muscular system). In everyday language, your aerobic endurance is your body's ability to use oxygen efficiently. Regular aerobic exercise makes all your activities seem easier to do, because the more conditioned you are, the better your body can take in and use oxygen.

To give you an example of the benefits of aerobic exercise, let's look at your heart. The heart is a muscle. In pumping blood, it delivers oxygen to all parts of your body (since oxygen travels through the bloodstream), including your other muscles. Muscles need a certain amount of oxygen to do a particular job, such as climb stairs, and your heart will have to do a certain amount of work to deliver the oxygen needed.

Like any other muscle, the heart will grow (hypertrophy) when trained properly. As your heart grows, it is able to pump more blood each time it beats, and with each beat, more oxygen is sent throughout your body. Over time, your heart won't have to work as hard to deliver the amount of oxygen needed for your other muscles to do a particular job. What that means in terms of your exercise program is this: with regular aerobic exercise, your heart will not have to work as hard as before to perform the same amount and intensity of exercise.

Aerobic Exercise and You

The decision of how and when to introduce aerobic exercise into your training will depend on several factors, including the following:

- Your current treatment status (You should not begin aggressive aerobic training while undergoing chemotherapy or radiation therapy. However, a self-paced walking program, in which you are not trying to keep your heart rate up in a "training zone"—explained on page 185—is appropriate and may help with nausea and fatigue.)

- Whether you were aerobically active before your breast cancer treatment
- Whether you have any other medical conditions that affect your ability to exercise, such as osteoporosis or heart disease

Ask your health care providers to help you assess your readiness for aerobic training.

Resuming Your Aerobic Training

If you were aerobically active before your breast cancer treatment, you probably already have an idea of which aerobic activities you like best and what level of intensity you want to achieve. Just remember that you cannot pick up where you left off. It is important to resume training at a low intensity and to progress gradually. This is true even if you are returning to aerobic exercise after completing some or all of the essential exercises in Chapter 4. Aerobic training places different demands on your body than flexibility and strength exercises, and your body needs time to adapt to these new demands. Hopefully, you are able to begin a self-paced walking program or perform some type of low-level aerobic exercise during or soon after your treatment.

The same basic safety suggestions that apply to all exercise training apply to aerobic exercise. Review "Points to Remember When Performing All Exercises" on page 46 and "Warning Signs to Stop Exercising" on page 35.

If you were active before surgery, there's no reason you should not be able to resume some type of aerobic activity as soon as your doctor gives you the OK. Low-level aerobic exercise in combination with flexibility exercises can generally begin almost immediately after surgery depending on how you feel. However, we suggest that you not begin the strength training in Levels II, III, and IV until you are at least six weeks after surgery, have completed the Level I exercises, and have met the progression criteria in the "At-Home Physical Assessment Sheet" on pages 42–43. You can warm up and stretch before doing your aerobic training, or you can move right from your warm-up into your aerobic training. You should then do your stretching exercises. This will prepare your body for the challenges of the strength training portion, which will come next. Finish with a proper cooldown, to allow your body to return to its pre-exercise state, and stretching.

Starting Aerobic Training for the First Time

If you were not aerobically active before your breast cancer treatment, now is a great time to start. Begin at a low level of exercise and progress slowly and gradually until you reach a level, and an appropriate stage in your recovery, to begin progressing more rapidly and working a little harder and longer. Eventually, you may get to the point where you are interested in maintaining—not increasing—your level of aerobic fitness.

Over just a few months, your heart and lungs will become stronger. You will have more energy, and everyday tasks will seem easier to do. And just think what your aerobic exercise program will mean. Not only will you be a breast cancer survivor, but many of you will be doing something you've never done before and will have made yourself even stronger than you were before breast cancer.

Many newcomers think that aerobic exercise means "aerobics class"—something that takes place at a health club, with rhythmic music playing and an instructor leading the way. In fact, any activity that gets your heart and lungs working harder than they normally do at rest and keeps them working hard for twenty minutes or more is aerobic exercise. Walking, swimming, bicycling, and many other common activities can be done aerobically.

If you were physically capable of doing a particular aerobic activity before your treatment—even if you weren't actually participating on a regular basis—you should be able to do that activity after treatment. Of course, you must start slowly and progress gradually, while carefully monitoring your response to any new exercise. And as always, get permission from your doctor before you begin.

Benefiting from Your Exercise Program

We have mentioned that many common activities, such as walking and biking, are aerobic activities when done at a level that sufficiently raises your heart rate for a minimum of twenty minutes. An important thing to remember, however, is that there is walking and there is *walking*. Although just getting up and moving is extremely important and has health benefits, you need to push yourself into your "training zone" to make real progress in improving your fitness level.

It is important to note that pushing yourself and working in your training zone are appropriate only after you have completed your treatment, have had your lab values evaluated, have been cleared by your doctor, have established an initial base of conditioning, and feel up to it. You can begin low-level activity, such as self-paced walking, during treatment, but you should not begin pushing yourself until you are ready. The recommendations for aerobic conditioning at the end of this chapter can help you begin your program.

Figuring out your training zone involves doing some simple arithmetic. You'll find the formula later in this chapter, in the section called "The FITT Principle" beginning on page 184. Monitoring yourself to make sure you stay in your zone during exercise can be as easy as taking your pulse or rating your exertion level.

So get ready to get fit. Break out the towels and make sure you drink plenty of water. It's extremely important that you replenish the water your body is losing through perspiration. Drinking plenty of water also will help rid your body of impurities and prevent you from becoming dehydrated.

Since exercise is going to be a big part of your life, you need to select activities that you will enjoy doing (or at least can tolerate) on a regular basis. Don't limit yourself to just one exercise. Select several items from your "exercise buffet" so that you won't get bored with the same old thing. (Exercises are discussed individually in the next section, "Examples of Aerobic Exercise.")

Variety not only keeps you interested in exercising but also challenges your body in different ways so that you continue to see and feel results. After you've been performing a certain exercise for a prolonged period, your body acclimates itself to that exercise. At that point, you will most likely reach a plateau, meaning that you will cease to make any further progress in weight loss, aerobic capacity, muscle growth, or strength gains. To get past a plateau, you can change your primary exercise altogether or just change the style and intensity of the exercise. Let's say, for example, that you are currently walking on a treadmill for thirty minutes at 0 percent incline and a speed of three miles per hour. To change your exercise, you could switch to a stationary bicycle. Or to change the intensity, you could increase the incline or the speed of the treadmill.

Another obstacle that many of you will encounter is maintaining your program while traveling. If you travel regularly, pick a primary exercise that you can do anywhere. This makes walking and stair climbing good choices for many people. No matter where you are, you can find a hallway or a flight of stairs.

Aerobic training is not a substitute for flexibility and strength training. You need to continue your *Essential Exercises* program after you begin aerobic training. The general safety suggestions for aerobic training are the same as for other types of exercise. If you haven't already done so, now is a good time to review "Points to Remember When Performing All Exercises" on page 46, and "Warning Signs to Stop Exercising" on page 35.

Examples of Aerobic Exercise

Most of the exercise activities discussed in this section require little special equipment. For many of the exercises, all you need is a pair of athletic shoes with good support and some comfortable, loose-fitting clothing. For others, the required equipment, such as a stationary bicycle, will be provided by the gym or health club where you exercise or may be available for purchase for use in your home. Most of the activities can be done on neighborhood streets or sidewalks, in your home, or in public facilities near your home. Selecting an activity will be your own personal choice, as some may be considered risky in light of your treatment. Be sure you understand all of the potential risks posed by the activities discussed in the following sections before you choose what to do.

Walking, Jogging, "Dancing," and Climbing

Walking is probably the most popular form of aerobic exercise and may be the best choice for you. You already know how to do it, you can do it just about anywhere, and, best of all, it's free. Another great thing about walking is that it puts much less stress on your muscles, ligaments, and joints than high-impact activities such as jogging or traditional aerobic dance.

Walking is a great first-step aerobic activity, and you can often start it immediately after surgery (with your doctor's permission). Pumping your arms as you walk burns more calories and pumps the lymphatic fluid through your affected arm. But be extremely careful not to aggravate your surgery wound by pumping too soon or too much. Walking with your arms at your sides is adequate exercise for most women after surgery.

You may choose to progress from walking to jogging, but this is not highly recommended. Jogging places a great deal of stress on the muscles, ligaments, and joints and commonly leads to overuse injuries of the knees and ankles. If you are prone to these injuries or have trouble with your hips or lower back, you should avoid jogging. If you are overweight by more than twenty pounds, it's important for you to lose some weight before trying to jog, because the extra weight will add even more stress to your joints.

If you feel that you have to increase your intensity from walking, you may want to try walk-jogging—walking for a while, then jogging for a while. Or try power-walking up hills. Walking up hills is extremely challenging and will certainly get you out of a slump.

In Chapter 2, we discussed the impact that breast cancer surgery can have on your posture. When you are walking or jogging, it is critical to maintain proper posture. Keep your head straight, chin up, and eyes looking forward.

One of the most enjoyable forms of exercise is aerobic dance, commonly called simply aerobics. Some of you may disagree, especially if you have two left feet (or two right ones), but don't worry; this is not dancing in the Fred Astaire–Ginger Rogers sense. Aerobic dance is the activity many people automatically think of when they hear the term *aerobic exercise.* These aerobics classes have come a long way from the high-impact classes of the 1980s. A good instructor will pace the class according to the fitness level of the participants. Some classes are more challenging than others with respect to both the energy level required and the fancy footwork involved. The key is to find a class or two that you really enjoy.

These days, there are hip-hop, funk, box aerobics, Afro-Brazilian, water aerobics, step, slide, and kickboxing classes, to name just a few. You certainly won't get bored with any of these classes. If you choose to participate, make sure you observe every caution and understand all the potential risks. Aerobics and the many variations available today may pose some additional risks for you in light of your treatment. Bouncing, punching, kicking, stepping, and sliding pose risks for falling and jerking your arm. Be aware that, as a result of these activities, you could injure your arm, shoulder, or surgical site, or possibly get lymphedema. By contrast, these activities, when done carefully and under control, can be extremely empowering and great stress relievers. It is your personal decision whether or not to participate in the different activities in light of the potential risks.

As with jogging, aerobic dance has been associated with a multitude of overuse injuries. If you already suffer from knee or lower back problems, you will probably want to avoid high-impact and step aerobics classes. Otherwise, if you keep your jumping and bouncing to a minimum, you should remain injury-free.

Climbing stairs is another great aerobic exercise. It is certainly affordable, and you should be able to find a flight of stairs nearby. Surprisingly, many people find it very difficult to climb a long flight of stairs. As with any other activity, the more often you do it, the easier it becomes. If you want to be efficient at climbing stairs, you will need to climb a lot of stairs. Many of you will find yourselves breathless before you reach the top. Take the "talk test": If you can carry on a conversation while you are climbing stairs (or doing any other exercise), you are more than likely exercising at an appropriate level. If you can't talk and are huffing and puffing your way to the top, you're working too hard.

Skiing and Swimming

Skiing and swimming, depending on how they are done, may be slightly less aerobic than the activities mentioned above, but what they lack in aerobic benefit, they make up for in fun. Although skiing is contingent on the weather and is expensive (lift tickets, transportation, lodging, and gear), many people enjoy it. If you can tolerate the cold and love to be outside, skiing is absolute bliss.

You have two choices when it comes to skiing: For you daredevils and thrill seekers, downhill skiing is the thing. For those seeking fewer risks, lower costs, and easier access, cross-country skiing is the answer. Please understand that both cross-country and downhill skiing may be more dangerous than other activities. You should have a clear understanding of the risks involved.

Cross-country skiing is highly aerobic and trains both the upper and lower body. It places little stress on your joints, because you remain in contact with the ground at all times. If you're new to the sport, you may find it a little challenging at first because of the balance and coordination required. If you have undergone breast surgery, you'll definitely want to clear cross-country skiing with your doctor. This activity requires a great deal of upper body strength, endurance, and repetitive motion. You will also need to have fairly good range of motion. Doing the strength training exercises in this book may help prepare you for the physical demands of skiing.

Downhill skiing doesn't require nearly as much upper body strength as cross-country skiing, but the chances of falling are much greater, and thus put you at a greater risk for injury. It is critical that you receive your doctor's permission before trying downhill skiing. You also need to take great care when you are on the slopes. Although you will seldom have a choice of which side to fall on, if you can, try to fall on your unaffected side.

Perhaps the sound of island music and the smell of ocean air are more appealing to you. If so, swimming is certainly an option. Swimming is a moderately aerobic activity and is one of the safest and least stressful of all exercises. It is the perfect exercise following breast surgery to help you get the full range of motion back in your arm and shoulder without placing too much stress on the joints. If you had a latissimus dorsi flap, you may have to wait a little longer for your incision to heal so that you can swim pain-free. Swimming may be an excellent way for you to start an exercise program during your initial recovery. If you are currently undergoing chemotherapy or radiation, you must receive your doctor's approval prior to swimming. Most likely you will have to wait until that treatment is done.

Bicycling and In-line Skating

Bicycling and in-line skating are moderate aerobic activities that are great fun and allow you to enjoy the outdoors. Unfortunately, both activities carry with them a very high injury rate from falls and other accidents. It may be wise to wait a few months after surgery before attempting these activities. Although the activities themselves require mainly leg strength, you will undoubtedly rely on your arms to break a fall. And a fall, especially on your affected arm, could result in cuts or scrapes, muscle or connective tissue damage, or even broken bones. These injuries could lead to infection and/or an inflammatory response, which could cause lymphedema. If you fall on your affected arm, tend immediately to any cuts or scrapes or musculoskeletal injuries. Make sure that you contact your physician.

Give yourself ample time to recover from surgery before taking to your wheels. Find a bicycle path or other route with little or no traffic. Although you may feel like a space creature with all that protective gear, make sure you wear it. You're not in a fashion show, and those crazy little plastic and foam gadgets could save your life.

As with downhill skiing, you'll spend a good part of your time going downhill. Although that part may prove to be the most fun, you will do the least work and get the least aerobic benefit from it. But don't discount the psychological benefit of being outside on a beautiful day. Also, biking and in-line skating are great ways to spend time with friends and family.

If you don't want to take the chance of falling on an outdoor bike, you may want to try spinning. Available at many gyms and health clubs, spinning takes place in a room filled with stationary bikes. Spinning classes are high energy, and instructors use visualization to take you on a guided tour through outer space, the wine country, or anywhere else they feel like traveling. You need to be in somewhat good shape to participate, because these classes are grueling. Spinning is probably one of the most intense workouts you will ever do, but it can be safe, effective, and fun if you follow basic precautions.

When biking, whether indoors or outdoors, avoid gripping the handlebars tightly and leaning heavily on them. This places stress on your affected arm and can raise your blood pressure. Keep your weight centered and on the seat as much as you can.

Other Options

Currently, one of the hottest exercise crazes is Pilates. Similar to yoga in many ways, the Pilates program allows you to refine your body awareness and increase your balance, strength, and flexibility. Pilates is not an aerobic exercise, but we feel that it deserves a mention here. Both Pilates and yoga are fantastic choices after surgery to help you regain your range of motion and flexibility in a safe and comfortable environment (with modification to the exercises where necessary).

Sports such as basketball, handball, racquetball, and tennis are often more recreational than aerobic. Don't count them as your regular aerobic activity unless your skills and fitness level let you really go at it and push yourself hard. These activities can be dangerous in terms of potential injury to your affected arm.

Interval Training

Interval training can be applied to most forms of aerobic activity and is used by many competitive athletes. It often involves periods of maximum, or near-maximum, effort (you're basically working as hard as you can), followed by short periods of rest. Because of the high intensity, only well-trained individuals should do maximum or near-maximum intervals. An untrained person who attempts these is at increased risk of injury, not to mention rapid fatigue.

Another type of interval training involves fitness intervals, in which you increase the intensity of your exercise for brief periods during your workout. You are encouraged to push yourself a little harder for two to three minutes and then return to the lower intensity. For example, if you were on a treadmill walking at a speed of three miles per hour with a 0 percent incline, you might increase your speed to three and a half miles per hour and your incline to 3 percent. You would stay at the more challenging level for two to three minutes, or until you became breathless, and then return to the original intensity. Fitness intervals help you add variety and intensity to your program.

Whatever exercise or activity you choose, talk with your health care providers and assess the risks associated with it before you begin. Knowing the possible dangers of an exercise will allow you to participate as safely as possible by taking as many precautions as you can.

The FITT Principle

"FITT" stands for frequency (how often you exercise), intensity (how hard you exercise), type (what kind of exercise you do), and time (how long you exercise). When using these variables to construct your exercise program, it is imperative that you do the correct type of exercise in the correct way to get the desired results. In other words, exercise is specific.

For example, if running is your main exercise and you're the fastest runner in town, you may decide to take up stair climbing as a new challenge, assuming that you will be an excellent stair climber as well. But, to your surprise, you can't make it to the top of the stairs without gasping for air. How can this be? Indeed, to be good at a specific sport or task, you need to train for that sport or task. Different sports rely on different muscle groups and energy systems.

Let's break the FITT principle down so that it is easy to understand.

Frequency

This refers to the number of days per week that you engage in a particular aerobic activity. The rule of thumb is that you should do the activity a minimum of three times per week. If you are not quite ready (physically or emotionally) to handle three times per week, do as much as you can comfortably. As you progress with your exercise program, and depending on your individual goals, you may find it necessary to increase the number of days per week. Make sure you allow yourself adequate time for rest and recovery between exercise sessions to minimize the risks associated with overtraining.

Intensity

The intensity of an exercise is a critical component. Exercise at too high an intensity will require your body to use the anaerobic energy system (without adequate oxygen), causing you to breathe harder, have difficulty talking, and tire quickly. In this situation, you won't be able to exercise for very long.

You want to exercise at as high an intensity as you can without getting too winded. Take the "talk test": can you carry on a conversation without losing your breath? If the answer is no, slow down.

The optimum intensity for cardiovascular fitness improvement is 60 to 90 percent of your maximum heart rate (maximum heart rate equals 220 minus your age). For example, the estimated maximum heart rate for a 40-year-old woman would be 220 minus 40, or 180. Her optimum training range, or training zone, would be 60 to 90 percent of 180, or 108 to 162. This range may seem a little broad, but it's appropriate, because many other factors are considered when determining an individual's exercise intensity range. These factors include age, current level of fitness, health history, medications, and weight, among others. Also, some people are more "genetically gifted" than others and are able to perform at higher intensities.

The maximum heart rate method for determining exercise intensity is not foolproof. Several things can either raise or lower your heart rate, including caffeine, alcohol, cold medicine, blood pressure medication, stress, and illness. It is best to use the Borg Rating of Perceived Exertion (RPE) Scale along with your heart rate to make sure that you are exercising at the proper intensity. This subjective method measures how hard you feel that you are exercising on a scale of 6 to 20 (see below). Think of level 6 as sleeping peacefully, level 11 as walking at a regular pace (light), level 15 as walking as fast as you can up a steep hill (hard), and level 20 as so hard that you must stop (maximal exertion). For most people, exercising at a level of 13 (somewhat hard) to 15 (hard) correlates well with an appropriate training zone.

Rating of Perceived Exertion Scale

6 No exertion at all	**11** Light	**16**
7 Extremely light	**12**	**17** Very hard
8	**13** Somewhat hard	**18**
9 Very light	**14**	**19** Extremely hard
10	**15** Hard (heavy)	**20** Maximal exertion

Borg, RPE scale © 1970, 1985, 1994, 1998. Reprinted with permission. *For correct usage of the RPE scale see the instructions and administration found in Borg, G. Borg's Perceived Exertion and Pain Scales. Chapmaign, IL: Human Kinetics, 1996.

Remember that when you are just getting started, the important thing is to get up and get moving. As you continue to build your stamina and strength, you can begin to think about your intensity.

Type

Type refers to the kind of exercise you are doing. For example, to achieve maximum effectiveness in aerobic training, the exercise needs to be rhythmical and continuous and to involve large muscle groups. Walking, jogging, cycling, stair climbing, and aerobic dance all satisfy these criteria. Activities involving both upper and lower extremity movements—such as cross-country skiing, rowing, swimming, and box aerobics—also lead to increased aerobic capacity and better total body conditioning.

Time

Time refers to how long you exercise. Aerobic exercise must last at least twenty minutes per session at your target heart rate to lead to substantial cardiovascular fitness improvement over time. If you increase your intensity, you can decrease the duration to achieve a similar training effect. The twenty-minute rule works very well for most women following breast surgery. You may need to start your aerobic exercise by alternating short intervals of exercise at your target rate with intervals at a lower intensity until you can do fifteen to twenty minutes at your target rate. This approach is also generally effective for those who are new to exercise programs, seniors, and obese persons.

If you have already been exercising on a regular basis, you will probably need to train a bit longer to see continued improvement. A good recommendation is a minimum of three aerobic sessions per week, each lasting thirty to forty-five minutes.

If one of your goals is to lose weight, aerobic exercise might help. If you want to keep weight off, aerobic exercise is essential. For weight loss, exercising aerobically five or six times per week will certainly be more effective than exercising three times per week. But you must always take into account how you are feeling and adjust your program accordingly.

Suggestions for Beginning Your Aerobic Program

When you begin an aerobic exercise program, start slowly and proceed patiently. Remember to record your activity and your thoughts in your exercise journal (see page 39). Warm up, cool down, and stretch as part of every exercise session. Consult "Points to Remember When Performing All Exercises" on page 46. And, as always, consult your physician before beginning any exercise program.

Aerobic Exercise (FITT)

FREQUENCY   Progress to 3 times per week. After your aerobic capacity improves, aim for 3–5 times per week.

INTENSITY   Aim for 50–75% of maximum heart rate for unsupervised or initial aerobic training. (If you are currently undergoing treatment, follow a self-paced walking program and do not worry about a "training zone." If just starting training, begin at the low end of the training range.) With improved aerobic fitness, aim for a range of 60–85% of maximum heart rate. An example of a good target heart range for general conditioning would be walking or cycling at 70–75% of 220 minus your age. RPE should be 11–14.

TYPE   Exercise that involves continuous, rhythmical movements of large muscle groups are recommended: walking, swimming, or cycling (stationary or outdoor cycling, but be very cautious not to fall on or injure your affected side).

TIME   Begin aerobic training with an interval program in which 3–5 minutes of exercise (for instance, walking or cycling) is performed at your target heart rate, followed by either 1–2 minutes of exercise at a lower heart rate (slower pace) or 1–2 minutes of rest. If the exercise intervals at the target heart rate are too difficult, reduce the time in the training zone and increase the lower-intensity (or rest) intervals. Progress by increasing the exercise minutes and decreasing the rest period. When you can complete 15 minutes of continuous exercise, begin to work up to 30 continuous minutes by adding 2–4 minutes of exercise time per week. (Refer to the next section, "Final Notes," for instructions on how to progress slowly and gradually.)

Final Notes

As mentioned previously, you need to think about your aerobic conditioning as a progression:

- Start slowly and at a very low level (particularly if you are still undergoing treatment) and listen to your body. Don't worry about your training zone or pushing yourself.

- As you feel better and are cleared by your doctor, begin to build an initial base of conditioning. Work a little harder and try to stay at the lower end of your training range (40 to 65 percent). Go by how you feel and progress gradually.

- If you feel ready and the doctor says OK, try adding some intervals of harder work to your program. Use the intervals to help you establish a base that lets you do 15 minutes of continuous activity, then build to 30 minutes.

- If you are already pretty fit and can already do 30 straight minutes, go by how you feel and work at a level at which you are comfortable.

- Note that if you are on any medications that affect your heart rate, the heart rate training zone will not be accurate. In this case you can monitor your progress by RPE.

- Modify your exercise according to your stage of treatment and recovery, your current fitness level, other medical concerns, and your personal goals.

CHAPTER 6

Weight Training

While the well-known regimen of surgery/radiation/chemotherapy treats breast cancer, *Essential Exercises* . . . documents that carefully planned, regular physical exercise treats the treatment. It allows women to regain their former selves, and in some cases, find improved levels in their quality of life.

Bonnie Goldstein, Breast Cancer Survivor
Producer, "Cancer in the Family," ABC News Documentary

All experience is an arch to build upon.   —*Henry Adams*

THERE IS A GREAT DEAL OF CONTROVERSY about lifting weights after breast surgery. If you speak with ten different doctors, you will most likely get ten significantly different opinions. This can drive even the most sane exercise enthusiast a bit crazy. The problem is that there has not been enough empirical research in this area to provide conclusive evidence as to the positive or negative effects of weight training on post–breast surgery patients. The use of exercise in this population is relatively new and most often has been limited to aerobic exercise and flexibility training.

Although only a limited amount of research has focused specifically on women recovering from breast cancer, we do know that patients who exercise have shown improvements over those who do not exercise in functional capacity, body composition, nausea, mood, fatigue, sleep, and self-esteem. One example of this can be found at the Santa Barbara Athletic Club in Santa Barbara, California, where the exercise program for cancer patients includes a weight training circuit. The program has produced average upper body strength increases of 35 percent and improvements in general quality of life. Another example is the Breast Cancer Physical Therapy Center in Philadelphia, which employs a comprehensive exercise program for lymphedema associated with breast cancer. The program consists of flexibility training, aerobic exercise, and progressive weight training.

Before beginning a weight training program, you must seek the advice and permission of your doctor. If your doctor does not give you the green light or does not advocate weight training, you may want to get opinions from other doctors in the field. There may be a very legitimate reason for you to avoid weight training. If so, you will need to find alternative forms of exercise.

The key is to use caution and not to lift weights that are too heavy, especially in the beginning. If you were an avid weight lifter prior to your surgery and you haven't experienced any complications, there is no reason you can't continue your weight training regimen, as long as no contraindications develop. However, your progression must be slow and gradual.

Surgery and Weight Training

Depending on the type of surgery you had, certain restrictions may be placed on which muscle groups you can use and the degree to which you can use them. See Chapter 2 for a detailed discussion of surgical procedures and their impact on the body. Following is some information specifically related to weight training.

In breast-conserving surgery only the tumor and varying amounts of surrounding breast tissue are removed. Some lymph nodes may be removed as well. When the incision has healed properly, there should be virtually no limitations on what you can do. On average, healing takes six weeks. You should regain normal or close to normal range of motion before beginning to lift weights. Use caution so that you don't irritate your incision. Start with light weights (one to two pounds), and if you don't experience any negative effects after your first few sessions—particularly in regard to your arm—gradually increase your weights. Lymphedema is a possible side effect of axillary lymph node dissection and radiation, so progress slowly and carefully if these were part of your treatment.

In a simple mastectomy, only breast tissue is removed. If you allow your body enough time to heal, you should experience no limitations in your weight training program.

A modified radical mastectomy includes removal of the breast and some of the axillary lymph nodes. The main chest wall muscles are left intact. Following surgery, you may experience some tightening of the chest wall. In this early stage, the emphasis should be on range-of-motion exercises rather than lifting weights. Good range of motion is critical before you begin a weight training program. As your range of motion improves and you experience no other complications, begin adding weights to your routine. Because of the lymphedema risk associated with axillary lymph node dissection, be cautious in your progression.

If you had reconstructive surgery, you must be more cautious about your weight training routine. For example, if you had a latissimus dorsi flap, you can expect a longer recovery time and a little more discomfort than with an implant or expander. As we noted in Chapter 2, the "tunneling" that is done to move tissue from the back to the breast will disturb a lot of other tissue along the way.

If the tissue is taken from your abdomen in a TRAM flap, you will no longer have the same strength in your abdominal muscles, and you may have difficulty performing sit-ups. Because your abdominal muscles will be weakened, you may be more prone to lower back problems. It is then extremely important to protect your back and practice back safety and proper lifting techniques. Do not perform any sit-ups or lifting activities until you have permission from your doctor.

If the tissue is taken from your back and not your abdomen, postoperative healing will be quicker. There is still the potential for weakening of the back and shoulder area, and you may need more physical therapy. A number of women suffer from stiffness and pain after a latissimus dorsi flap, because it alters the balance of the entire shoulder area. This highlights one of the biggest concerns for weight training—muscular balance. When you have an imbalance between the strength of particular muscle groups, it can make you more prone to injury. A good example would be someone who has very weak abdominal muscles and a fairly strong back. Although the back is strong, it has to work twice as hard to support the torso because of the weak abdominal muscles, and the extra strain on the back means that there is a much greater chance of back injury. Also, because flap procedures can affect your posture, you will want to pay particular attention to strengthening the supporting muscles in your weight training program. These include your upper back and shoulder girdle muscles (including the rhomboids, serratus anterior, middle and lower trapezius, and rotator cuff muscles).

As with any surgical procedure, the more complicated the reconstructive surgery, the longer the recovery time, the greater the number of possible side effects, and the slower your weight training progression should be. But don't be discouraged; be patient. Treat your body with lots of love and care. You have been through a lot and need a little nurturing.

Regardless of the type of reconstruction you have had, if at any time you feel excessive discomfort or pain in the affected area, stop exercising immediately and seek the advice of your doctor. Also, if you notice any swelling in your arm, consult your physician immediately.

Your Weight Training Program

Before you begin each weight training session, it is imperative that you do at least a five-minute warm-up. The warm-up should consist of any type of *aerobic* activity that will increase your heart rate and body temperature. It may include walking, jogging, biking (stationary or outdoors), or stair climbing. The warm-up should be slow and gradual to prevent any sudden rush of blood to the arms and legs. It is one of the most important aspects of your workout and should not be skipped. It prepares the muscles for more vigorous activity by allowing a gradual redistribution of blood to the working muscles. This redistribution of blood has a warming effect on the muscles, which increases the elasticity of the connective tissue and other muscle components. These changes may reduce the risk of injury to your muscles, tendons, and ligaments.

As we discussed in Chapter 4, you can follow your warm-up with stretching. Stretching will help increase your joints' range of motion and may reduce the risk of injury to tight muscles. Each stretch should be held for a minimum of ten to thirty seconds. Avoid forceful bouncing motions, which can actually cause injury. You will want to pay particular attention to the chest and shoulder areas and devote a little extra time to stretching those muscles, whether or not they were directly affected by your surgery. After warming up and stretching, you are ready to begin your weight training program. (And remember—always stretch again when you are done.)

Make sure that you don't lift too heavy a weight or do too many repetitions. Standard guidelines for strength training in the general healthy population suggest that if an individual cannot do 8–12 repetitions with a given weight, that weight is too heavy and should be reduced. Alternatively, if the individual is able to do more than 12 repetitions with ease, the weight is too light and should be increased. Standard guidelines have not yet been established for breast cancer survivors, but anecdotal evidence suggests that weight training should begin with one- to two-pound weights and progress much more gradually and slowly than a program for someone who is not at risk for lymphedema.

The affected arm's response to the exercise is used to determine the appropriateness of the intensity. That is, you should not experience any swelling or change in tissue texture in the affected arm. If you do, stop exercising and contact your physician. When you're given the OK to continue, reduce the intensity and volume of your workout. The goal is to begin with 8–10 repetitions and build up to two or three sets of 8–12 repetitions. You should never work at a level where your arm and shoulder area feel achy or heavy while you're lifting weights. Overdoing it can cause strains or sprains, which can trigger an inflammatory response and possibly lymphedema.

Weight training can be combined with aerobic interval training (see page 183), in which you perform short aerobic intervals to elevate your heart rate, then keep your heart rate elevated with weight training intervals. This should only be done with professional guidance to ensure that a proper and controlled pace is maintained. You must also be at an appropriate level of conditioning.

After starting your weight training program, you may notice that the scale indicates that you have gained weight. Don't be discouraged. Muscle weighs more than fat. Lean muscle is good; it burns more calories than fat, and having more muscle increases your overall metabolism. If you take two women who weigh 150 pounds and one has 18 percent body fat and the other 30 percent, the one with 18 percent will probably be wearing a size smaller than the one with 30 percent. This is because she has all that good lean muscle. It weighs more but is tighter, firmer, and healthier.

Work on perfecting your weight training form at your own pace. The idea is to discover your own path to the next level of fitness. Don't settle for making yourself as strong as you were before; try to make yourself stronger.

Remember to record your activity and your thoughts in an exercise journal (see page 39). Always warm up, cool down, and stretch. Refer to "Points to Remember When Performing All Exercises" on page 46. And, as always, consult your physician before beginning any exercise program.

FIRMS Strength Training

The acronym to remember for weight training is FIRMS: frequency, intensity, repetitions, muscles, and sets.

Frequency

Exercise two or three times per week with at least one day of rest in between weight training sessions.

Intensity

Begin with an exercise band (follow the precautions discussed in Chapter 3) or one- to two-pound weights; the weight should allow you to work up to 8–10 consecutive repetitions. After tolerance in the affected arm is established, use a weight that allows 8–12 repetitions, and continue to progress to heavier weights that keep you in the 8–12 range (see "Repetitions" and "Sets" below). Do not increase the weight more than 5 percent each time you increase your intensity. Progress more slowly and gradually than if you had not been treated for breast cancer. Do not work through feelings of achiness or heaviness. (If using a band, hold it so that the resistance allows you to perform the appropriate number of repetitions.)

Repetitions

When beginning weight training, work up to performing 8–10 repetitions per exercise. After your tolerance to exercise is established, progress to 8–12 repetitions per exercise.

Muscles

Exercise all the major muscle groups: arms, chest, back, shoulders, buttocks, legs, and abdominals.

Sets

Begin with one set of each exercise and progress to two or three sets.

References

CHAPTER 1

American College of Sports Medicine. *ACSM's guidelines for exercise testing and prescription.* 6th ed. Baltimore: Lippincott Williams & Wilkins, 2000.

———. *ACSM's resource manual for guidelines for exercise testing and prescription.* 3rd ed. Baltimore: Williams & Wilkins, 1998.

———. *Exercise management for persons with chronic diseases and disabilities.* Champaign, Illinois: Human Kinetics, 1997.

Bernstein, L., B. E. Henderson, and R. Hanisch, et al. Physical exercise and reduced risk of breast cancer in young women. *Journal of the National Cancer Institute* 86(18):1403–1408, 1994.

Segar, M., et al. Aerobic exercise reduces depression and anxiety and increases self-esteem among breast cancer survivors (abstract). *Medicine and Science in Sports and Exercise* 27(5S):S212, 1995.

———. The effect of aerobic exercise on self-esteem and depressive and anxiety symptoms among breast cancer survivors. *Oncology Nursing Forum* 25(1):107–113, 1998.

Thune, I., et al. Physical activity and the risk of breast cancer. *New England Journal of Medicine* 336(18):1269–1275, 1997.

U.S. Department of Health and Human Services, Centers for Disease Control and Prevention, National Center for Chronic Disease Prevention and Health Promotion. *Physical activity and health: A report of the surgeon general.* Atlanta: U.S. Department of Health and Human Services, 1996.

U.S. Department of Health and Human Services, National Center for Health Statistics. *Healthy people 2000 review, 1995–96.* Hyattsville, Md.: Public Health Service, 1996.

Winningham, M. L., M. G. MacVicar, M. Bondoc, J. I. Anderson, and J. P. Minton. Effect of aerobic exercise on body weight and composition in patients with breast cancer on adjuvant chemotherapy. *Oncology Nursing Forum* 16(5):683–689, 1989.

World Cancer Research Fund/American Institute for Cancer Research. *Food, nutrition, and the prevention of cancer: A global perspective.* Washington, D.C.: American Institute for Cancer Research, 1997.

CHAPTER 2

Aaronson, Naomi. Designing classes for breast cancer survivors. *Idea Today* (May):55–61, 1997.

American Cancer Society. Reach to recovery: Exercises after mastectomy patient guide. http://www.cancer.org, 1983.

American College of Sports Medicine. *ACSM's guidelines for exercise testing and prescription.* 6th ed. Baltimore: Lippincott Williams & Wilkins, 2000.

———. *ACSM's resource manual for guidelines for exercise testing and prescription.* 3rd ed. Baltimore: Williams & Wilkins, 1998.

———. *Exercise management for persons with chronic diseases and disabilities.* Champaign, Illinois: Human Kinetics, 1997.

Baron, R. Sensory alterations after breast cancer surgery. *Clinical Journal of Oncology Nursing* 2(1):17–23, 1998.

Brinker, N. G., and C. McEvily Harris. *The race is run one step at a time.* Arlington, Texas: Summit Publishing Group, 1995.

Brown, D. Personal interview. Women's Exercise Research Center, Exercise Science Program, School of Public Health and Health Services, George Washington University, 1997, 1998.

Cox, C., and D. Reintgen. Reply to lymphatic mapping and sentinel node biopsy in breast cancer. *JAMA Letters* 277:791–792, 1997.

Dollinger, B., E. H. Rosenbaum, and G. Cable. *Everyone's guide to cancer therapy: How cancer is diagnosed, treated, and managed day to day.* Toronto: Somerville House Books, 1994.

Durak, E. P., and P. C. Lilly. Cancer rehab in the health club. *Fitness Management* (February):30–32, 1997.

Friedewald, V., and A. U. Buzdar with M. Bokulich. *Ask the doctor: Breast cancer.* Kansas City, Missouri: Andrews & McMeel, 1997.

Giuliano, A. E. Lymphatic mapping and sentinel node biopsy in breast cancer. *JAMA Letters* 277:791, 1997.

Giuliano, A. E., R. C. Jones, M. Brennan, and R. Statman. Sentinel lymphadenectomy in breast cancer. *Journal of Clinical Oncology* 15:2345–2350, 1997.

Groenwald, S. L, M. H. Frogge, M. Goodman, and C.H. Yarbro, eds. *Cancer nursing: Principles and practice.* 4th ed. Boston: Jones & Bartlett, 1997.

Halverstadt, A. A survey: Exercise in women with breast cancer. Master's thesis, Exercise Science Program, School of Public Health and Health Services, George Washington University, May 1998.

Karakousis, C. P., et al. The technique of sentinel node biopsy (abstract). *European Journal of Surgical Oncology* 22(3):271–275, 1996.

Kisner, C., and L. A. Colby. *Therapeutic exercise: Foundations and techniques.* 2nd ed. Philadelphia: F. A. Davis, 1990.

MacVicar, M. G., and M. L. Winningham. Promoting functional capacity of cancer patients. *Cancer Bulletin* 38:235–238, 1986.

MacVicar, M. G., M. L. Winningham, and J. L. Nickel. Effects of aerobic interval training on cancer patients' functional capacity. *Nursing Research* 38(6):348–351, 1989.

Memorial Sloan-Kettering Cancer Center. Kinder, gentler breast surgery. http://mskcc.org/patients_n_public/about_cancer_and_treatment/cancer_information_by_type/breast_cancer/kinder_gentler_breast_surgery_.html, 1997.

Miaskowski, C. *Oncology nursing: An essential guide for patient care.* Philadelphia: W. B. Saunders, 1997.

National Cancer Institute. http://www.nci.nih.gov/.

New England Medical Center. NEMC's breast health center offers new treatment options. Press Release 97121501, December 15, 1997.

Otto, S. E. *Oncology nursing.* 3rd ed. St. Louis: Mosby, 1997.

Reintgen, D. What is the role and impact of the sentinel node sampling technique in breast cancer staging? *Cancer Control Journal* 4(3), (Supplement), May/June 1997. On-line journal. http://www.moffitt.usf.edu/cancjrnl/.

Reintgen, D., et al. The role of selective lymphadenectomy in breast cancer. *Cancer Control Journal* 4(3), May/June 1997. On-line journal. http://www.moffitt.usf.edu/cancjrnl/.

Saccone, S. Recovering from breast cancer: Fitness programs can help empower women to heal more quickly in body and mind—here's how to start one. *Idea Today* (June):26–30, 1995.

Small, W., and M. Morrow. Local management of primary breast cancer. *Cancer Control Journal* 4(3), 1997. On-line journal. http://www.moffitt.usf.edu/cancjrnl/.

Stalheim-Smith, A., and G. K. Fitch. *Understanding human anatomy and physiology.* St. Paul: West Publishing Company, 1993.

Stumm, D. *Recovering from breast surgery.* Alameda, Calif.: Hunter House, 1995.

Veronesi, U., G. Paganelli, V. Galimberti et al. Sentinel-node biopsy to avoid axillary dissection in breast cancer with clinically negative lymph nodes—can axillary dissection be avoided in breast cancer? *Lancet* 349:1864–1867, 1997.

Winningham, M. L. Exercise in breast cancer rehabilitation: Exploring new horizons. *Innovations in Oncology Nursing* 7:1–14, 1992a.

———. Role of exercise in cancer therapy. In *Exercise and disease,* ed. R. Watson and M. Eisinger. Boca Raton, Fla.: CRC Press, 1992b.

———. Walking program for people with cancer: Getting started. *Cancer Nursing* 14:270–276, 1991.

Winningham, M. L. and M. G. MacVicar. The effect of aerobic exercise on patient reports of nausea. *Oncology Nursing Forum* 15(4):447–450, 1988.

Winningham, M. L., M. G. MacVicar, M. Bondoc, J. I. Anderson, and J. P. Minton. Effect of aerobic exercise on body weight and composition in patients with breast cancer on adjuvant chemotherapy. *Oncology Nursing Forum* 16(5):683–689, 1989.

Winningham, M. L., M. G. MacVicar, and C. A. Burke. Exercise for cancer patients: Guidelines and precautions. *The Physician and Sportsmedicine* 14(10):125–134, 1986.

CHAPTER 3

Aaronson, Naomi. Designing classes for breast cancer survivors. *Idea Today* (May):55–61, 1997.

American College of Sports Medicine. *ACSM's guidelines for exercise testing and prescription.* 6th ed. Baltimore: Lippincott Williams & Wilkins, 2000.

———. *ACSM's resource manual for guidelines for exercise testing and prescription.* 3rd ed. Baltimore: Williams & Wilkins, 1998.

———. *Exercise management for persons with chronic diseases and disabilities.* Champaign, Illinois: Human Kinetics, 1997.

Brown, D. Personal interview. Women's Exercise Research Center, Exercise Science Program, School of Public Health and Health Services, George Washington University, 1997, 1998.

Durak, E. P. and P. C. Lilly. Cancer rehab in the health club. *Fitness Management* (February):30–32, 1997.

Howley, E. T., and B. Franks. *Health fitness instructor's handbook.* 3rd ed. Champaign, Illinois: Human Kinetics, 1997.

Kisner, C., and L. A. Colby. *Therapeutic exercise: Foundations and techniques.* 2nd ed. Philadelphia: F. A. Davis, 1990.

MacVicar, M. G., and M. L. Winningham. Promoting functional capacity of cancer patients. *Cancer Bulletin* 38:235–238, 1986.

MacVicar, M. G., M. L. Winningham, and J. L. Nickel. Effects of aerobic interval training on cancer patients' functional capacity. *Nursing Research* 38(6):348–351, 1989.

Miaskowski, C. *Oncology nursing: An essential guide for patient care.* Philadelphia: W. B. Saunders, 1997.

Saccone, S. Recovering from breast cancer: Fitness programs can help empower women to heal more quickly in body and mind—here's how to start one. *Idea Today* (June):26–30, 1995.

Segar, M., et al. Aerobic exercise reduces depression and anxiety and increases self-esteem among breast cancer survivors (abstract). *Medicine and Science in Sports and Exercise* 27(5S):S212, 1995.

———. The effect of aerobic exercise on self-esteem and depressive and anxiety symptoms among breast cancer survivors. *Oncology Nursing Forum* 25(1):107–113, 1998.

Stumm, D. *Recovering from breast surgery.* Alameda, Calif.: Hunter House, 1995.

Winningham, M. L. Exercise in breast cancer rehabilitation: Exploring new horizons. *Innovations in Oncology Nursing* 7:1–14, 1992a.

———. Role of exercise in cancer therapy. In *Exercise and disease,* ed. R. Watson and M. Eisinger. Boca Raton, Fla.: CRC Press, 1992b.

———. Walking program for people with cancer: Getting started. *Cancer Nursing* 14:270–276, 1991.

Winningham, M. L., and M. G. MacVicar. The effect of aerobic exercise on patient reports of nausea. *Oncology Nursing Forum* 15(4):447–450, 1988.

Winningham, M. L., M. G. MacVicar, M. Bondoc, J. I. Anderson, and J. P. Minton. Effect of aerobic exercise on body weight and composition in patients with breast cancer on adjuvant chemotherapy. *Oncology Nursing Forum* 16(5):683–689, 1989.

Winningham, M. L., M. G. MacVicar, and C. A. Burke. Exercise for cancer patients: Guidelines and precautions. *The Physician and Sportsmedicine* 14(10):125–134, 1986.

CHAPTER 4

Aaronson, Naomi. Designing classes for breast cancer survivors. *Idea Today* (May):55–61, 1997.

American College of Sports Medicine. *ACSM's guidelines for exercise testing and prescription.* 6th ed. Baltimore: Lippincott Williams & Wilkins, 2000.

———. *ACSM's resource manual for guidelines for exercise testing and prescription.* 3rd ed. Baltimore: Williams & Wilkins, 1998.

———. *Exercise management for persons with chronic diseases and disabilities.* Champaign, Illinois: Human Kinetics, 1997.

Brown, D. Personal interview. Women's Exercise Research Center, Exercise Science Program, School of Public Health and Health Services, George Washington University, 1997, 1998.

Durak, E. P., and P. C. Lilly. Cancer rehab in the health club. *Fitness Management* (February):30–32, 1997.

Howley, E. T., and B. Franks. *Health fitness instructor's handbook.* 3rd ed. Champaign, Illinois: Human Kinetics, 1997.

Kisner, C., and L. A. Colby. *Therapeutic exercise: Foundations and techniques.* 2nd ed. Philadelphia: F. A. Davis, 1990.

Saccone, S. Recovering from breast cancer: Fitness programs can help empower women to heal more quickly in body and mind—here's how to start one. *Idea Today* (June):26–30, 1995.

Segar, M., et al. Aerobic exercise reduces depression and anxiety and increases self-esteem among breast cancer survivors (abstract). *Medicine and Science in Sports and Exercise* 27(5S):S212, 1995.

———. The effect of aerobic exercise on self-esteem and depressive and anxiety symptoms among breast cancer survivors. *Oncology Nursing Forum* 25(1):107–113, 1998.

Stumm, D. *Recovering from breast surgery.* Alameda, Calif.: Hunter House, 1995.

Winningham, M. L. Exercise in breast cancer rehabilitation: Exploring new horizons. *Innovations in Oncology Nursing* 7:1–14, 1992a.

———. Role of exercise in cancer therapy. In *Exercise and disease,* ed. R. Watson and M. Eisinger. Boca Raton, Fla.: CRC Press, 1992b.

———. Walking program for people with cancer: Getting started. *Cancer Nursing* 14:270–276, 1991.

Winningham, M. L., and M. G. MacVicar. The effect of aerobic exercise on patient reports of nausea. *Oncology Nursing Forum* 15(4):447–450, 1988.

Winningham, M. L., M. G. MacVicar, M. Bondoc, J. I. Anderson, and J. P. Minton. Effect of aerobic exercise on body weight and composition in patients with breast cancer on adjuvant chemotherapy. *Oncology Nursing Forum* 16(5):683–689, 1989.

Winningham, M. L., M. G. MacVicar, and C. A. Burke. Exercise for cancer patients: Guidelines and precautions. *The Physician and Sportsmedicine* 14(10):125–134, 1986.

CHAPTER 5

American College of Sports Medicine. *ACSM's guidelines for exercise testing and prescription.* 6th ed. Baltimore: Lippincott Williams & Wilkins, 2000.

———. *ACSM's resource manual for guidelines for exercise testing and prescription.* 3rd ed. Baltimore: Williams & Wilkins, 1998.

———. *Exercise management for persons with chronic diseases and disabilities.* Champaign, Illinois: Human Kinetics, 1997.

Brown, D. Personal interview. Women's Exercise Research Center, Exercise Science Program, School of Public Health and Health Services, George Washington University, 1997, 1998.

Durak, E. P., and P. C. Lilly. Cancer rehab in the health club. *Fitness Management* (February):30–32, 1997.

Howley, E. T., and B. Franks. *Health fitness instructor's handbook.* 3rd ed. Champaign, Illinois: Human Kinetics, 1997.

Kisner, C., and L. A. Colby. *Therapeutic exercise: Foundations and techniques.* 2nd ed. Philadelphia: F. A. Davis, 1990.

Noble, B. J., G.A.V. Borg, I. Jacobs, R. Ceci, and P. Kaiser. A category-ratio perceived exertion scale: Relationship to blood and muscle lactates and heart rate. *Medicine and Science in Sports and Exercise* 15:523–528, 1983.

Winningham, M. L. Exercise in breast cancer rehabilitation: Exploring new horizons. *Innovations in Oncology Nursing* 7:1–14, 1992a.

———. Role of exercise in cancer therapy. In *Exercise and disease,* ed. R. Watson and M. Eisinger. Boca Raton, Fla.: CRC Press, 1992b.

———. Walking program for people with cancer: Getting started. *Cancer Nursing* 14:270–276, 1991.

Winningham, M. L., and M. G. MacVicar. The effect of aerobic exercise on patient reports of nausea. *Oncology Nursing Forum* 15(4):447–450, 1988.

Winningham, M. L., M. G. MacVicar, M. Bondoc, J. I. Anderson, and J. P. Minton. Effect of aerobic exercise on body weight and composition in patients with breast cancer on adjuvant chemotherapy. *Oncology Nursing Forum* 16(5):683–689, 1989.

Winningham, M. L., M. G. MacVicar, and C. A. Burke. Exercise for cancer patients: Guidelines and precautions. *The Physician and Sportsmedicine* 14(10):125–134, 1986.

CHAPTER 6
American College of Sports Medicine. *ACSM's guidelines for exercise testing and prescription.* 6th ed. Baltimore: Lippincott Williams & Wilkins, 2000.

———. *ACSM's resource manual for guidelines for exercise testing and prescription.* 3rd ed. Baltimore: Williams & Wilkins, 1998.

———. *Exercise management for persons with chronic diseases and disabilities.* Champaign, Illinois: Human Kinetics, 1997.

Durak, E. P., and P. C. Lilly. Cancer rehab in the health club. *Fitness Management* (February):30–32, 1997.

Kisner, C., and L. A. Colby. *Therapeutic exercise: Foundations and techniques.* 2nd ed. Philadelphia: F. A. Davis, 1990.

MacVicar, M. G., and M. L. Winningham. Promoting functional capacity of cancer patients. *Cancer Bulletin* 38:235–238, 1986.

Miaskowski, C. *Oncology nursing: An essential guide for patient care.* Philadelphia: W. B. Saunders, 1997.

Miller, L. T. The enigma of exercise: Participation in an exercise program after breast cancer surgery.

Saccone, S. Recovering from breast cancer: Fitness programs can help empower women to heal more quickly in body and mind—here's how to start one. *Idea Today* (June):26–30, 1995.

Segar, M., et al. Aerobic exercise reduces depression and anxiety and increases self-esteem among breast cancer survivors (abstract). *Medicine and Science in Sports and Exercise* 27(5S):S212, 1995.

Winningham, M. L. Exercise in breast cancer rehabilitation: Exploring new horizons. *Innovations in Oncology Nursing* 7:1–14, 1992a.

———. Role of exercise in cancer therapy. In *Exercise and disease,* ed. R. Watson and M. Eisinger. Boca Raton, Fla.: CRC Press, 1992b.

Winningham, M. L. and M. G. MacVicar. The effect of aerobic exercise on patient reports of nausea. *Oncology Nursing Forum* 15(4):447–450, 1988.

Winningham, M. L., M. G. MacVicar, and C. A. Burke. Exercise for cancer patients: Guidelines and precautions. *The Physician and Sportsmedicine* 14(10):125–134, 1986.

Resources

THIS RESOURCE LIST has been compiled from many sources but is by no means all-inclusive. We think all the listings should be helpful, although we are not personally familiar with every one of them. Most of these agencies can provide information in Spanish as well as English. Even if they can't answer your questions, they will refer you to the right place.

American Cancer Society

1599 Clifton Road NE, Atlanta, GA 30329-4251, 800-ACS-2345, www.cancer.org

Call for cancer-related pamphlets and other materials at your local ACS unit or state-chartered division. If you are unable to obtain material locally, contact the ACS National Office at the address or phone number listed above.

Look Good, Feel Better

800-395-LOOK,
www.lookgoodfeelbetter.org

Founded in 1989 and developed by the Cosmetic, Toiletry, and Fragrance Association in partnership with the American Cancer Society and the National Cosmetology Association, this program is designed to help women recovering from cancer deal with various changes in their appearance associated with cancer treatment. Call for referrals to free workshops hosted by hair and makeup professionals. Brochures and information are in English and Spanish.

Reach to Recovery

800-ACS-2345

The American Cancer Society trains cancer survivors to meet and talk with breast cancer patients on a volunteer basis. A volunteer will generally go to the hospital to visit the patient after surgery to help with a prosthesis or to talk about reconstruction. Typically, the volunteer has gone through the same type of procedure or treatment as the patient. Reach to Recovery also offers support groups for lumpectomy and mastectomy patients.

American Society of Plastic and Reconstructive Surgeons

444 East Algonquin Road, Arlington Heights, IL 60005, 800-635-0635, www.plasticsurgery.org

Will provide you with a list of board-certified plastic and reconstructive surgeons by geographic area and an educational brochure in about a week's time. You can also find out whether a particular physician is board certified and/or a member of the society.

Breast Cancer Physical Therapy Center

1905 Spruce Street, Philadelphia, PA 19103, 215-772-0160

For $8.95, the center will send you a booklet on exercises to help manage lymphedema.

Breast Cancer Survivors Foundation

P.O. Box 1050, Lake Oswego, OR 97034, www.Breastcancersurvivors.com

Founded in 2000, this organization is an information resource and provider of grants and outreach programs.

Cancer Wellness Center

Barbara Kassel Brotman House, 215 Revere Drive, Northbrook, IL 50062, 708-509-9595

Offers free emotional support on its 24-hour hot line and through support groups, relaxation groups, educational workshops, and a library.

Corporate Angel Network Inc.
Westchester County Airport, 1 Loop Road, White Plains, NY 10604, 914-328-1313, www.corporateangelnetwork.org

A nationwide program designed to give cancer patients seats on corporate aircraft traveling to and from recognized treatment centers. There is no financial need requirement or cost to the patient.

Edith Imre Foundation for Loss of Hair
30 West Fifty-seventh Street, Second floor, New York, NY 10019, 212-757-8160

Provides counseling, support, and wig selection.

ENCORE
Sponsored by the YWCA, this program for postoperative breast cancer patients includes exercise to music, water exercises, and a discussion period. With your doctor's permission, you can join the third week after surgery. For more information, contact the YWCA in your area.

Komen Alliance
Susan G. Komen Breast Cancer Foundation, 5005 LBJ Freeway, Occidental Tower, Suite 370, Dallas, TX 75244, 800-I'M AWARE, www.breastcancerinfo.com

Will send you information on screening, BSE, treatment, and support, as well as the booklet *Caring for Your Breasts*. This organization provides a comprehensive program for research, education, and the diagnosis and treatment of breast disease.

**National Alliance
of Breast Cancer Organizations**
9 East Thirty-seventh Street, Tenth floor, New York, NY 10016, 212-719-0154, E-mail: nabcoinfo@aol.com

NABCO provides a multitude of resources for both patients and health care professionals. It publishes an annual Breast Cancer Resource List, which includes comprehensive listings of all of the services available from nearly three hundred support groups across the nation. The cost is $3. It also publishes a periodic newsletter for members, which includes fact sheets on treatment and research.

National Cancer Institute
800-4-CANCER, www.cancer.gov

The primary federal agency for cancer research and information on everything from research projects to new treatments and drugs. It provides cancer-related pamphlets and other materials and includes the Cancer Information Service.

National Lymphedema Network Hotline
1611 Telegraph Avenue, Suite 1111, Oakland, CA 94612, 510-208-3200
800-541-3259, www.lymphnet.org

A nonprofit organization that provides patients and professionals with information about prevention and treatment of lymphedema, a side effect of lymph node surgery. You can request an information packet with referrals for medical treatment, physical therapy, general information, and support in your area.

Y-ME National Hotline
212 West Van Buren Street, Chicago, IL 60607, 800-221-2141, www.y-me.org

Provides lists of both national and regional hot lines, as well as referrals for medical care and support groups. Trained volunteers are matched by background and experience to callers. The organization also has a wig and prosthesis bank for women who cannot afford these items.

Glossary

Abduction   Movement away from the midline of the body. An example would be a leg lift to the side that works your outer thigh.

Adduction   Movement toward the midline of the body. An example would be bringing your legs from a straddle position to a closed parallel position.

Adjuvant therapy   Additional treatment used after cancer surgery that focuses on preventing the cancer's return.

Adriamyacin   A strong chemotherapy drug used for metastatic breast cancer.

Aerobic exercise   Activities in which the oxygen demands of the muscles are met by the oxygen supplied by the heart and lungs. Typical aerobic exercises are aerobic dance, bicycling, jogging, walking, and other activities that use large muscle groups.

Anaerobic exercise   Activities in which the oxygen demands of the muscles are so high that the body cannot supply enough oxygen. "All-out" activities such as sprinting and weight lifting are examples.

Anemia   A condition marked by an abnormally low number of circulating red blood cells or hemoglobin concentration. Symptoms include tiredness, shortness of breath, and weakness.

Anorexia   Loss of appetite.

Antioxidants   Enzymes that help clean up the hazardous waste our bodies produce. This waste, known as free radicals, is made up of molecules and often sets the stage for cancer. You can keep antioxidant levels high by consuming ample amounts of beta-carotene and vitamins A, C, and E. Talk to your doctor about appropriate amounts to consume.

Atrophy   A reduction in the size of tissue or muscle mass, usually resulting from prolonged periods of inactivity, bed rest, or disuse.

Axilla   Armpit.

Axillary lymph node dissection   Surgical removal of some of the lymph nodes under the arm. If the original biopsy reveals invasive cancer, this procedure may be performed at the time of the lumpectomy or mastectomy. The lymph nodes are then evaluated to see whether the cancer has broken through or is still contained in the nodes.

Bilateral   Affecting both sides of the body.

Body composition   Relative amounts of muscle, bone, and fat in the body.

Breast implant   A prosthetic device placed under the skin after the breast is removed. Typically, a silicone bag filled with saline (salt water).

Calcium   An important body mineral that is vital to the development and maintenance of bone.

Calorie   See *kilocalorie*.

Cardiovascular fitness   The ability to perform moderate- to high-intensity exercise for prolonged periods of time without undue fatigue.

Chemotherapy   The treatment of cancer by drugs designed to kill the cancer cells and stop them from growing.

Circumduction   Circular motion of a limb.

Connective tissue   Tissue that binds, supports, or separates specialized tissues or organs.

Cooldown   Exercise intended to allow the body—especially heart rate, blood pressure, and temperature—to gradually return to a resting state. It is suggested that the cooldown last ten to fifteen minutes and involve the same muscle groups as the main exercise.

Cruciferous vegetables   Vegetables such as broccoli, cauliflower, and brussels sprouts that are high in beta-carotene and are thought to help protect against some types of cancer.

Diabetes   A condition caused by the body's inability to produce enough insulin or to use insulin properly.

Dynamic exercise   Alternate contraction and relaxation of a muscle or group of muscles causing either a partial or complete movement throughout the joint's range of motion.

Dysphagia   Difficulty swallowing. Food may seem to be stuck in the throat. This can be a side effect of some breast cancer treatments.

Dyspnea   Shortness of breath.

Edema   The accumulation of fluid in tissue; swelling.

Electrolytes   Chemicals such as sodium, bicarbonate, potassium, and chloride that are found in blood and tissue.

Estrogen receptor   Protein found on some cells to which estrogen molecules attach. If a tumor tests positive for estrogen receptors, it is sensitive to hormones. In women whose tumors are sensitive to hormones, a hormonal treatment can be used as adjuvant therapy.

Exhale   To expel air or vapor; breathe out.

Extension   The straightening of a limb. Opposite of *flexion*.

Fatigue   The point at which your cardiovascular endurance or muscles become exhausted and strength is diminished.

Flexibility   Range of motion possible in a joint or series of joints.

Flexion   The bending of a limb. Opposite of *extension*.

Free flap   Breast reconstruction wherein the tissue is removed and the feeding artery and vein are cut. The tissue is then moved to the location of the mastectomy incision, and the artery and vein are sewn to the artery and vein in the armpit.

Free radicals   Molecules making up the hazardous waste our bodies produce through everyday activity. These radicals can set the stage for cancer.

Frozen shoulder   Painful stiffness of the shoulder that makes it difficult to lift the arm over the head.

Heart rate   Number of beats (contractions) of the heart per unit of time; expressed as beats per minute.

Heat cramps   Involuntary cramping in muscles during exercise in the heat. This is often the result of an alteration of the sodium and potassium levels in the muscle due to dehydration and salt depletion.

Heatstroke   A condition resulting from the body's failure to regulate its core temperature. This is a medical emergency characterized by high body temperature; hot, usually dry skin; confusion; or unconsciousness.

Hormonal therapy   A form of cancer therapy that takes advantage of the tendency of some cancers to shrink or stabilize if certain medications are administered.

Hot flashes/flushes   Sudden sensations of heat and swelling associated with menopause.

Hypertension   Higher than normal blood pressure. Often defined as a resting blood pressure greater than 140/90 mm Hg.

Hypertrophy   Increased size of a muscle or other organ.

Hyperventilation   Deep and rapid breathing that can cause dizziness and other symptoms.

Inflammation   A defense mechanism of the body's tissue that causes extra white blood cells to pour into the tissue, leading to swelling, redness, heat, and pain.

Isometric An action of the muscle in which tension is developed but there is no shortening or lengthening of the muscle.

Kilocalorie (kcal) A measure of energy equal to the amount of heat required to change the temperature of 1 kilogram (kg) of water from 14.5 degrees Celsius to 15.5 degrees Celsius. Also called a calorie. A deficit of 3,500 kcal equals a 1-pound weight loss, whereas an increase of 3,500 kcal equals a 1-pound weight gain.

Kyphosis A condition of the back often referred to as hunchback; seen mostly in women after menopause.

Lactic acid Substance that forms in cells when glucose is metabolized in the absence of oxygen. For most, build-up results in fatigue.

Latissimus dorsi flap Flap of skin and muscle taken from the back (latissimus dorsi) and used for breast reconstruction after mastectomy.

Lordosis A condition of the lower back often referred to as swayback. There tends to be a flattening of the lordotic curve with age.

Lumpectomy Surgery to remove a cancerous lump without removing the entire breast. It is a less radical procedure than mastectomy and is usually followed by radiation.

Lymph nodes Oval glands found throughout the body that produce infection-fighting lymphocytes and filter out and destroy bacteria. They can be the body's first line of defense against the spread of cancer, as well as the location of cancer spread.

Lymphedema The swelling of the affected arm following surgery on the lymph nodes under the arm (axillary lymph node dissection). It can be either temporary or chronic and can occur immediately after surgery or at a later time.

Malignant Cancerous.

Margin A small "rim" of normal breast tissue around a tumor. In breast-conserving surgery, surgeons remove the tumor plus this rim, called the "margin of healthy tissue."

Mastectomy Surgery removing part of or all of the breast.

Menopause Final cessation of the menstrual cycle; change of life.

Muscular endurance The ability of a muscle or group of muscles to contract repeatedly at a submaximal force over time.

Muscular strength The maximal force generated by a muscle or group of muscles.

Neoadjuvant therapy Treatment used before other cancer treatments, generally to shrink the tumor by at least 50 percent before surgery is performed.

Obesity The accumulation and storage of excess body fat; the condition of being overweight. Obesity is an independent risk factor for the development of coronary artery disease. It is frequently the predecessor of type II diabetes.

Osteoporosis A condition that results in the loss of bone density and increases the risk of fractures and bone injuries. Most common in menopausal women. Weight-bearing exercise is recommended to counteract the effects of the disease and increase bone density.

Pallor Paleness.

Parallel Two lines or objects lying in the same, or nearly the same, direction without meeting or intersecting.

Perpendicular Two lines or objects meeting or lying at right angles.

Platelet One kind of blood cell. Platelets are responsible for creating the first part of a blood clot.

Prone Lying flat on one's stomach, face-down.

Radiation therapy   The use of high-energy radiation from X-ray machines, radium, cobalt, or other sources for the control or cure of cancer. It may be used to reduce the size of a tumor before surgery or to destroy any remaining cancer cells after surgery.

Rating of perceived exertion (RPE)   Numerical rating assigned to the perceived effort of an exercise task. Commonly known as the Borg Rating of Perceived Exertion Scale.

Red blood cell   One kind of blood cell. Red blood cells bring oxygen to tissue and take carbon dioxide from it.

Rehabilitation   Physical or emotional program that helps cancer patients adjust and return to a full and productive life.

Repetition   One complete execution of a particular motion in exercise.

Respiratory system   Bodily system that takes in and distributes the air we breathe so that blood high in oxygen and low in carbon dioxide can be pumped to all the cells.

Rotation   Turning.

Scar tissue   Thick, collagenous connective tissue laid down by the body in an attempt to repair injured tissue.

Sentinel node   The first lymph node in a cluster of nodes that drain a specific area of the body. In a procedure known as sentinel (lymph) node biopsy, the first node to receive lymph draining from the breast is identified and removed for examination. It is thought that since the sentinel node is the first to receive this fluid, it will be the node most likely to contain cancerous cells if they have spread from the primary site. If this node is found to be clear of cancerous cells, it is thought that the nodes past the sentinel node also will be clear of the disease.

Set   A group of repetitions of a certain movement or exercise.

Shoulder girdle   The shoulder blades (the two scapulae) and collarbones (the two clavicles). It is the attachment site for the five main muscles that provide dynamic stability to the scapulae.

Static exercise   The contraction of a muscle or group of muscles without movement of a joint. Also known as an isometric contraction.

Stroke volume   The volume of blood pumped from the heart with each beat.

Supine   Lying flat on one's back with the chin pointing upward.

Training zone   Heart rate that a person must achieve and maintain to improve cardiovascular fitness. Generally, 60 to 85 percent of maximum heart rate. Contingent on the physical state of the person doing the exercise.

TRAM flap   Transverse rectus abdominis myocutaneous flap. Procedure in which skin and muscle tissue from the abdomen are tunneled under the skin to the site of a mastectomy wound. The site on the abdomen is sewn closed. The tissue's feeding artery and vein remain attached so that the blood supply remains intact after the tissue is relocated.

Tumor   A cancerous or noncancerous lump, mass, or swelling.

Unilateral   On one side of the body.

Vertical   Directed perpendicularly to the plane of the horizon; upright.

Warm-up   A fifteen- to twenty-minute low-intensity cardiovascular exercise session that prepares the body for more rigorous activity and may prevent injury.

White blood cell   One kind of blood cell. White blood cells fight infection. Chemotherapy and radiation usually cause low white blood cell counts.

Index

About the Authors

Amy Halverstadt received her BA from Dartmouth College, her MA in international affairs from The George Washington University, and her MS in exercise science from The George Washington University. She conducted her exercise science master's thesis on exercise in women with breast cancer and received The George Washington University Graduate Exercise Science Academic Excellence Award. She is currently working on her Ph.D. in exercise physiology at the University of Maryland in order to further her career in research and teaching. Halverstadt is certified as a health and fitness instructor by the American College of Sports Medicine and as a personal trainer by the American Council on Exercise. Her work in the field has included developing fitness and quality-of-life programs for seniors, children, and breast cancer survivors, as well as working as a certified personal trainer. She also has served as the Governor's Appointee to the Oklahoma Governor's Council on Physical Fitness and Sports. In 1996, Halverstadt cofounded EM-POWER. In 1999, she taught human anatomy and physiology at The George Washington University. She currently lives in Washington, D.C., where she continues to run her own consulting business and works with other health professionals to empower breast cancer survivors through research, education, and exercise programming.

Andrea Leonard cofounded EM-POWER with Amy Halverstadt in 1996. She earned her BA from the University of Maryland in 1990 and continued her education to pursue a career as a personal trainer. She is certified as a conditioning specialist by the National Sports Performance Association, as a personal trainer by the American Council on Exercise, as a health and fitness instructor by the American College of Sports Medicine, and as a special populations expert by the Cooper Institute. Previously, she was director of personal training at the National Capital YMCA in Washington, D.C. Leonard founded and currently operates Leading Edge Fitness Consultants, an exercise and wellness consulting corporation, in which she continues to work with both healthy individuals and those with special needs. In January 2000, she relocated to West Linn, Oregon, with her husband, Scott, and son, Dylan. She dedicates herself to improving the lives of breast cancer survivors through a new, nonprofit organization that she recently cofounded, the Breast Cancer Survivors Foundation. The foundation was formed as an information source and provider of grants and outreach programs for those affected by breast cancer. You can learn more about the foundation at www.breastcancersurvivors.com.